Healing Back Pain N

The Mind-Body Program
Proven to Work

Arthur H. Brownstein, M.D., M.P.H.

Newleaf

Newleaf
an imprint of
Gill & Macmillan Ltd
Hume Avenue
Park West
Dublin 12
with associated companies throughout the world
www.gillmacmillan.ie

First published by Newleaf 2000
Copyright © 1999 by Arthur H. Brownstein
Published by arrangement with Harbor Press, Inc. All rights reserved.

ISBN-13: 978 07171 3015 3

Printed in Malaysia

This book is dedicated to all back pain sufferers,
and to the great Spirit of Life,
whose divine love can heal our greatest afflictions.

IMPORTANT NOTICE:

The ideas, positions, and statements in this book may in some cases conflict with orthodox, mainstream medical opinion, and the advice regarding health matters outlined in this book are not suitable for everyone. Do not attempt self-diagnosis, and do not embark upon any self-treatment of any kind without qualified medical supervision. Nothing in this book should be construed as a promise of benefits or of results to be achieved, or a guarantee by the author or publisher of the safety or efficacy of its contents. The author, the publisher, its editors, and its employees disclaim any liability, loss, or risk incurred directly or indirectly as a result of the use or application of any of the contents of this book.

Contents

= Foreword =

THE BOOK YOU ARE ABOUT TO READ has the potential to help you change your life in ways that go far beyond the relief of pain, to the healing of mind and soul. Dr. Brownstein's expertise is not only medical, but also deeply personal. He has visited the dark territory of pain, crawling on all fours to the toilet in the middle of the night because it hurt too much to walk. He's had the surgery, tried the drugs, felt the despair and the depression. And he has experienced his back pain as a gift, in fact as a blessing, because it has taught him about healing. Like many wounded healers, he has been gifted with a passion to pass on what he has learned to others. This book is his gift to you. Whether or not you have back pain, if you follow Dr. Brownstein's recommendations, you will have a longer, healthier, more loving and creative life.

I know how well Dr. Brownstein's program works because I offered a similar, if more general, program when I taught at Harvard Medical School and directed the Mind/Body Clinic at Boston's Beth Israel Hospital for most of the 1980s. I learned a lot about pain and healing from the people I was privileged to care for, as a silent partner in their trials, as well as a delighted recipient of their joys and insights.

I'll never forget Janna, an advertising executive who attended the clinic. She was beautiful, smart, and had been disabled with back pain on and off for several years. At 33, she felt as if her life was over. Her boyfriend walked out on her, and she lost her job. When repeated surgeries failed to provide relief, Janna turned to our program with great reluctance because it seemed too simple to help. How could learning to elicit what our Division Director, Herbert Benson, M.D., termed the relaxation response, learning to manage stress, eating a diet rich in fiber and low in processed foods, and practicing a systematic program of stretching based on hatha yoga possibly do what surgery could not? And yet, after ten weeks, Janna was nearly pain free. Furthermore, she felt that she was much more creative and energetic than she had ever been before. Even if the pain had persisted, she felt that she had learned a way of living that she might never have discovered were it not for the pain.

Healing comes from the Anglo-Saxon word *haelen*, which means wholeness. Most of us coast along in a state of relative unconsciousness and fragmentation until we face a serious challenge like illness. When we are suddenly stopped cold, unable to do the simplest things like bending over, straightening up, picking up a child or even a can of tomatoes, life is put in a new perspective. If the pain lasts long enough, it's like a little death. We are no longer who we were before, and we have not yet been reborn into who we will be. This period of uncertainty, this dark night of the soul, calls our most basic assumptions and values into question. Who are we, what is most valuable to us, and what is the meaning of a life well lived? These questions are part of the journey to healing, to wholeness. Whether or not we are cured physically like Janna, or still endure pain, healing is always possible. In fact, it is the most basic definition of emotional and spiritual growth.

Healing is a process of clarifying our values and changing our behaviors to reflect them. When the body is broken, health suddenly becomes precious and we take better care of ourselves. When we feel isolated in pain, we realize how blessed our family and friends are. We make time for them. When we can't work, we realize what we would most like to work at. We may even question our mortality. Are we just this body, or are we something more enduring? How do we nourish our spirits? If that nourishment comes from nature, music, art, play, or prayer, we learn to make time for that. The reward of healing is that we remember what is beautiful and valuable even if the pain goes away. We make our outside lives coherent with our inner values and we are whole.

Be gentle with yourself. Healing is a gradual process. Follow the excellent guidelines Dr. Brownstein has given you, working at your own pace, and find some allies in the process. No one heals alone. When we share our process, the difficulties as well as the triumphs, a kind of magic happens. In our communication with others, we learn and grow together.

And remember, healing is an adventure that can transform you forever not only physically, but emotionally and spiritually as well. Enjoy the journey!

Joan Borysenko
Boulder, Colorado

= Acknowledgments =

THE FOLLOWING PEOPLE have been instrumental in the creation of this book: Bert Holtje, my literary agent, Debby Young, my wonderful editor, Harry Lynn, my publisher, Indra Sharma, my father-in-law and master artist, Prof. M. Joshi, former Dean of Bombay University, School of Art, and Jim Abell, artist and writer.

I also wish to thank the following scientists, healers, and spiritual cheerleaders, who have contributed in one or more ways to my career path, my personal growth, and my inner healing: Dean Ornish, M.D., Lee Lipsenthal, M.D., Ben Brown, M.D., Ruth Marlin, M.D., Rob Saper M.D., Conrad Knudson, M.S., Hank Ginsberg, Werner Heibensteit, and the entire staff at the Preventive Medicine Research Institute in Sausalito, California, Larry Dossey, M.D., the late Norman Cousins, James E. Banta, M.D., former Medical Director of the Peace Corps during the Kennedy Administration and former Dean of Tulane University School of Public Health and Tropical Medicine, Edgar Mitchell, Ph.D., Apollo 14 Astronaut and Founder of the Institute of Noetic Sciences, Bernie Siegel, M.D., artist and chief healing assistant to God, Louise Hay, Bruno Cortis, M.D., spiritual cardiologist, Joan Borysenko, Ph.D., big sister and mentor, Marty Rossman, M.D., Steve Schwartz, M.D., Larry Payne, Ph.D., Founding President of the International Yoga Therapists Association, my Indian mentors in yoga: S. Kuvalyananda, S. Digambarji, Sri O.P. Tiwari, Vijayendra Pratap, Ph.D., and Dr. Sri Krisna, M.B.B.S., Ph.D., Frank Netter, M.D., medical illustrator, John Sarno, M.D., Mary Schatz, M.D., Robin McKenzie, Wendy Kahatsu, M.D., Andrew Weil M.D., David Simon, M.D., Medical Director of the Chopra Center for Well Being in La Jolla, California,

Gary Saldana, M.D., Rob Ivker, D.O., President of the American Holistic Medical Association, Len Wisneski, M.D., holistic endocrinologist, Tuck and Betty Craven, M.D., Richard Posoff, and all the wonderful doctors, teachers, and people who have healed me with their unconditional love.

To all my patients and staff at the Princeville Medical Clinic, and to my wife Nutan and son Shantanu Brownstein, for their unselfishness, patience, and support during the five years it took me to finish this book, I thank you sincerely.

= Introduction =

AS A FORMER BACK PAIN PATIENT, I am well aware of the intense physical pain that accompanies back problems. I am also aware of the deeper emotional and mental anguish that afflicts the spirit when debilitating back pain strikes.

We are presently in the midst of a huge global epidemic of back pain. According to the latest government figures, back problems are now the number one cause of disability in the United States for people under the age of 45, with upwards of $100 billion spent annually. Seven out of ten people in the U.S. will suffer serious back pain at some stage in their lives. In Europe, some reports say that the numbers may be even greater.

Despite the hundreds of books and abundant literature on back pain, the problem continues to escalate. Clearly, the problem of back pain is not being adequately addressed.

Additionally, because so many back problems occur on the job and lead to court cases, to avoid legal hassles, many orthopedic surgeons now refuse to see patients with back problems. Where is a patient with back pain to turn for help if the supposed experts refuse to get involved?

I have read nearly every back pain book published in the past 20 years in search of a solution to my own back pain. I have also treated patients from all over the world who come to my clinic in Hawaii with their back problems, after most of them have already consulted with other doctors prior to seeing me. In reading these books and talking to these patients, I am still appalled at how much wrong information is out there. No wonder people are so confused while the back pain epidemic continues to rage out of control.

Based on first-hand experience, this book was written to set the record straight and to clear up all the nonsense that currently exists about back pain. Although I am a doctor, the material comes from the perspective of my own healing as a chronic back pain patient.

One of the greatest misconceptions about back pain is that it can be traced to a single incident, accident, or injury. I have seen many back patients, including myself, attribute all their pain and suffering to a specific event, such as the car accident of June 12, 1985, or the construction job incident of April 4, 1979. While at first glance this may seem to be the case, the accident or injury is usually just a triggering event. It is the "straw that broke the camel's back." It is the tip of the iceberg of an unhealthy process that had been going on for months or even years. The bottom line is that there is almost always more going on behind the scenes in the form of stress, tension, and other factors that conspire against you to cause your back problems.

To focus only on the mechanical aspects of your back pain can keep you stuck on the surface, never allowing you to understand the deeper causes of your problem. This will interfere with your healing. It's like not knowing what's behind the walls or underneath the floors of the house in which you live. When you have a leak in your plumbing, you better know what's behind the walls if you want to fix the problem. The same holds true for your back.

Another misconception about back pain is that it can be successfully treated by doctors and surgeons. Back pain is often attributed to a specific anatomical problem or defect, such as a ruptured disc, a bone spur, a ligament tear, a crushed vertebra, or some other anomaly. Doctors are very good at producing the tests that may help you actually see these defects, pinpointing the problem in great detail. They can also perform sophisticated, precise surgical procedures that fix these defects and supposedly lead to a cure.

But the truth is, when these specific problems or defects have been identified and presumably repaired by surgery, in a majority of cases, the pain still persists.

And what is the standard treatment for this continued pain? Why more surgery, of course! With repeated surgeries, the pain increases and the condition of the back deteriorates further; with each surgery the body's natural anatomy is altered and further weakened. Even if the surgery is successful, if the underlying problems are not addressed, the pain will come back. Clearly, surgery is not the ultimate cure for back pain.

As a physician, I do not dispute the fact that specific defects in the back can exist and that they can be documented by diagnostic procedures such as MRI and CAT scans. I also do not dispute the fact that surgery can be very helpful in certain instances. However, to really get at the root of your back pain and find a deeper, longer-lasting cure, you need to ask yourself the following questions:

1. What caused the problem (defect) in the first place?

2. How do I know that the problem (defect) is responsible for my pain?

3. If the problem (defect) is causing my pain, is it permanent or can it be healed?

4. If the problem (defect) is not permanent and can be reversed or healed, how can I make the pain go away and heal my back at the same time?

A major premise of this book is that if you are in pain, you can be healed. This is because where there is pain, there is life. Another premise is that the majority of problems causing back pain can be reversed if you understand the underlying processes that created the problem and are willing to take the time to heal it. Of course, doing something about the problem when it first surfaces makes the healing easier and faster, but even if you've been through surgery, as I have, you can still heal your back. This book shows you how to do it, and how to prevent further problems from recurring.

After years of effort aimed at healing my own back pain, I developed a method that worked for me and has worked for thousands of my patients. I call it the Back To Life Program, and this book takes you through each step of the program in a way that makes it easy to understand and implement. It is based on safe and effective principles that combine the best of modern science with ancient mind-body healing techniques.

The first chapter describes my own personal healing journey through a painful back condition that persisted for years and included traumatic surgery. In it "the straw that broke the camel's back" is used as a metaphor to illustrate that you must understand and address your underlying problems in order to heal your back.

In the second chapter, you'll be introduced to the anatomy of your back to help you understand how your back functions. You'll learn why the muscles are the most important part of your back in maintaining a healthy spine, how the mind and muscles are connected by the nervous system, and how stress can directly harm your back. You'll become aware of the important role your mind plays in the health of your back.

In the third chapter, you'll learn why pain is an important message from your body. You'll discover how pain can be a valuable teacher, friend, and vehicle for healing. You will also learn how you can understand and work with your pain. You'll be introduced to important mind-body strategies that will help you ultimately overcome your pain.

In the fourth chapter, you'll learn gentle, soothing stretches that will make your body flexible and will help you directly relieve the pain from tight and tense back muscles.

Chapter Five provides guidelines for safe and simple exercises that will help strengthen, support, and fortify your back.

In the sixth chapter, you'll learn powerful and effective stress management techniques including deep relaxation, breathing, guided imagery, visualization, and meditation. Just a few minutes a day using these techniques will help you manage your stress, calm your nerves, relax the muscles in your back, and ease your pain.

In Chapter Seven, you'll learn about diet, nutrition, and helpful eating habits for a strong and healthy back. You'll learn which harmful substances to avoid and which natural supplements to take to strengthen your back and make it feel better.

Chapter Eight tells you how to go back to work after a back injury. Specific reconditioning exercises and stretches are prescribed for a variety of on-the-job activities, including sitting, stooping, bending, lifting, and driving. Practical preventive strategies to ensure a strong and healthy, pain-free spine for years to come are emphasized.

Chapter Nine deals with the healing qualities embodied in the spirit of play, and why play is important for your back. The therapeutic value of hobbies, sports, entertainment, vacations, and the practical benefits of maintaining a sense of humor are discussed.

In Chapter Ten, you'll be taken "behind the scenes" to explore the emotional and spiritual factors that affect the health of your spine. By examining the connections between your mind, body, and the emotional and spiritual dimensions of your life, you'll learn how to access the deeper realms of your being to promote your back's health and overall wellness.

In a final special section on emergency back care, you are given specific instructions to follow in the event of severe, incapacitating back pain of sudden onset.

The word *healing* comes from the Greek, meaning *to make whole*, and there are several important truths I've discovered about this word that I would like to share with you here at the outset:

1. What is going on in your life can affect the health of your spine.

2. You can heal your back and overcome your pain. To accomplish this, try to see your pain as a teacher, your body as a gift, your mind as an instrument of your healing, and yourself as a being much greater than your body or your mind. *The whole is greater than the sum of its parts.*

Even though dark clouds of despair may surround you as you begin to take your first steps on the road to healing, you will soon discover a glimmer of light that will grow in brightness. I too began my journey in the darkness and am now surrounded by light. The light is beautiful and it is real, and it is waiting for you.

CHAPTER ONE

The Straw That Broke the Camel's Back

"ART, YOU'RE TAKING THIS OPERATION too lightly", said Dr. Masferrer, my neurosurgeon. "I'm afraid you just don't understand. I'm going to break your back!"

It was July of 1986 and I was lying in bed at the U.S. Air Force Regional Medical Center with excruciating pain and numbness running down my right leg into my foot and toes. The myelogram, a special X-ray of the spine, showed a large disc rupture between the fourth and fifth lumbar vertebrae. After two weeks of bedrest with no let up in the pain and numbness, it was time to go in and operate.

How did I end up in this mess, me, a doctor of all people? Besides the pain, it was embarrassing to be a patient in my own hospital!

To my best recollection, my back trouble began when I was about 21 years old. I was still in school when I took a job loading and unloading trucks at a large warehouse to help support myself. I put in long, grueling days that involved a lot of lifting. It seemed like the "manly" thing to do, and besides, I was young and strong and enjoyed sweating and doing hard physical labor. I was at that age when I thought I was invincible. I never said no to work of any kind. In fact, I never said no to much of anything, and that, I discovered later, was a major drawback to the future health of my spine.

On the job, one of the games we played in our spare time was King of the Warehouse. In this test of male macho strength, we would stand at opposite ends of the warehouse, lower our shoulders, and charge at each other like human battering rams, trying to knock each other over. Having been a surfer and a football player, I had good balance, timing, and strength. Additionally, I loved contact sports.

My boss, Bob, at 6'5" and 305 lbs, loved to square off against me, even though he could never defeat me. As we charged from opposite corners of the warehouse like a couple of raging bulls, I would come up on him from underneath, flicking my shoulder and smacking into him at the last possible moment. Upon impact, Bob would be sent flying.

One day, however, while playing this game, things didn't quite work out right for me. As Bob and I squared off in opposite corners prior to charging, I was feeling a little tired. When we slammed into each other my timing was slightly off. I knocked him down anyway, but absorbed the entire force of the blow in my lower back. That night I went home feeling a little stiffer than usual.

The next day in chemistry lab at UCLA, while bending over to get my glassware from the bottom drawer of my desk, I felt an electric shock travel clear up through my neck and into my head. It was a sudden, jolting sensation. In an instant, my legs gave out beneath me as I found myself sitting on the floor with both feet splayed out in front of me. There was no strength in my legs whatsoever. Strangely, there was no pain either. I brushed myself off, stood up, and as there were no residual symptoms, I decided to continue on with my activities as if everything were fine. I completely dismissed the significance of this event. To this day, I have never told a soul, not even my doctors.

Less than two years later, while wheeling a half-ton operating room table into one of the operating rooms at UCLA, my back did something funny again. As I returned to a standing position after bending down, I found I couldn't straighten up all the way, as if someone had jammed a broomstick up my hind quarters. It was rather unnerving. "I certainly can't resume my duties in this condition," I thought to myself. I ducked into a vacant room and cautiously backed up to the side of another operating table. Reaching down with my arms, I forced myself into a backbend as far as I could go until I heard a "pop." Miraculously, my back had snapped back into proper alignment. I was both grateful and relieved to find that now I could straighten up and move without any restrictions. Once again I went back to work, resuming my normal duties as if nothing had happened.

Two years later, during my first year in medical school, I found myself alone and isolated in a strange city. Philadelphia, where I was now living, was experiencing its worst winter in 25 years. I was an hour and a half away from school by rail commute and the trains kept breaking down because of the deep snows and sub-zero temperatures. I was also in the middle of a strained relationship that eventually broke apart.

By itself, the first year in medical school is emotionally demanding. With these complications, however, my standing as a first year medical student was in serious jeopardy, especially since I couldn't get to class for lectures and labs. On the occasions that I did make it into school when the trains were running, I worked off the stress by playing basketball.

During one basketball game, while coming down for a rebound, my back went out just like it had done that day in the operating room two years before. This time, however, I couldn't straighten myself up and pop my back into place.

I showered and then grabbed my books and athletic bag with great difficulty. My body was stuck in a bent-over position. Hobbling to the curb outside of the medical school, I reasoned that if I could make it to the library across the street, perhaps my back would slip back into place on its own. I glanced up and saw an elderly woman crossing the street, slowly, but with ease. I was envious of her and at that moment, I felt very old. The bags I was carrying felt like they weighed two tons each. It was horrible to feel so helpless.

Somehow I made it to my seat in the library and while turning to my neighbor, Rob, who was also a medical student, I mentioned something about my back to him. Before I knew it, Rob had brought a wheelchair to my seat, insisting on wheeling me to the emergency room. As I reluctantly got in, I felt embarrassed being wheeled past all the other medical students, doctors, and nurses in the library.

In the emergency room, after a four-hour wait, I had X-rays taken. The orthopedic resident (doctor-in-training), after looking at the films in a back room, gave me all of two minutes of his time. He managed to tell me on his hurried way out of the examining room that despite my being bent over sideways and unable to straighten up, all that was wrong with me was a simple muscle strain. "But I'm sure I slipped a disc or something," I pleaded with the resident. "Then go to another orthopedic surgeon for a second opinion if you don't believe me," he said. In the midst of my pain and confusion, this was all he could offer me.

I refused to believe that all that was wrong with my back was a simple muscle strain. It was way too painful for that. As an athlete, I had experienced many muscle strains before. I had also separated both shoulders and had ruptured an inguinal hernia while lifting weights when I had the flu. I felt I wasn't a sissy and had a fairly good tolerance for pain. The diagnosis that the resident had given me, according to my understanding, did not correlate with my pain. I felt slighted. Either he was wrong, which I was determined to prove, or if he was right, then I was being a big baby about this whole thing. My mind was reeling at a hundred miles an hour trying to figure out what was going on with my body! Why was I in so much pain?

Dr. Hoffman, a professor of orthopedics at my medical school, had a private office not far from our school. He examined me briefly, reviewed my films, and concluded that it was possible that my disc had slipped. Inwardly, I was comforted that now my pain was justified with this more serious diagnosis. "You better take care of yourself or you're headed for an operation," he informed me. I didn't realize how prophetic his words were at the time.

I took a room near my medical school so I wouldn't have to deal with the hassles of the lengthy rail commute and the inconsistent trains. Unable to walk without support, I hobbled to class on a pair of crutches through the snow.

I phoned my father, a psychiatrist at the UCLA School of Medicine, and told him what had happened. "Are you under stress?" he asked. "Dad, I was coming down from a rebound while playing basketball.

What the hell does stress have to do with it?!" I retorted angrily. It would take me 15 more years of back problems before I would realize the accuracy of my father's line of questioning.

After about a month, my back slowly improved. With this incident, however, I could no longer ignore my back. I needed to make some changes in my life if I wanted to avoid back surgery.

I enrolled in a yoga class to help bring some flexibility to my body and, in particular, to help me avoid the possibility of surgery. I also needed to deal with the anxiety of medical school and to learn how to relax and manage my stress. My yoga teacher assured me that if I were a sincere and regular student, all of these things were possible. While practicing yoga for the next five years, the condition of my back improved tremendously, and I did learn how to relax.

There were several setbacks during this period, however, as my back went out at inopportune times during periods of accumulated stress. The triggering events were physical traumas that while sometimes severe, could also be quite minor. One time my back went out lifting two full five-gallon water bottles, another time while wrestling with a friend, still another while bending down to pull on a boot. There seemed to be no correlation between the degree of trauma and the severity and duration of the pain. One thing seemed true, however; each time my back went out, it took longer to heal, and this had me worried.

In September of 1983 I entered the Air Force and was sent to the Philippines on active duty as payback for a military scholarship I was awarded during medical school. In this physically demanding environment, I ran 4-6 miles a day, swam 1,000 meters a day, biked 20-25 miles a day, and surfed 5-10 hours every weekend to maintain a warrior's level of fitness. For three full years, I participated in helicopter rescue missions and did extensive flying all over the Far East without any back problems whatsoever.

In May of 1986 however, dark, ominous clouds appeared on my horizon. My mother, brother, and father had all passed away in the last three years, and my wife at the time was at home dying of cancer, where I was trying to take care of her.

We had just purchased an expensive piece of property in Hawaii. The political climate of the Philippines was tense as the Marcos regime was ready to fall. The military was preparing for conflict. It was all too much, and like the proverbial straw that broke the camel's back, my back went out as well.

To take my mind off my problems, I had flown down to a remote outer island with some friends. On the airplane ride back home, while merely turning around to talk to the person in the seat behind me, my back began to stiffen. After an hour or so, I was locked in a death-grip of painful back muscle spasms and could barely shuffle my way off the plane.

With my back out, I tried to give it rest. The military, however, ordered me back to work. This added to the underlying tensions of being incapacitated. So once again I went into my familiar denial mode, put on a back brace, swallowed some pills, and tried to ignore the pain as I reported back to work like a good soldier.

My back was making its own efforts to heal, but the improvements were too slow for the fast pace of the Air Force. I felt pressured for time. I tried to accelerate the healing process with anything I could get my hands on — pills, electronic devices such as infra-red lamps, TENS (transcutaneous electrical nerve stimulators), heating pads, traction devices, hanging boots, braces, balms, and plenty of other stuff.

Sitting is the worst thing for an injured back, and having to man my desk for eight hours on end did not help my situation. As a member of the military, there was also the constant stress of war readiness, having to respond to contingencies on short notice.

In the previous three years, when my back had shown improvement, surfing had helped me overcome stress. I headed out to the ocean practically every weekend with a few buddies. Now, however, with my painful back, I found that I was unable to surf. I wondered how I would be able to manage my stress.

After more than a month, as stress kept building, I was eager to get back in the water. My back was still pretty bad, but the call of the ocean and the waves was strong.

On a chance visit to Base Operations, headquarters for all flight operations including the latest weather information, I saw a satellite photo of a huge typhoon that was heading our way. I could tell from the storm's size and direction that the waves were going to be good on the weekend. I couldn't resist. I decided to go surfing.

After a three-hour drive, when I finally got to the beach, my back was stiff and sore. I had no right to be there, but in my sheer pig-headed stupidity, I told myself that this would be good for me. As I carried my board to the water's edge, I told myself that I would be careful once I was in the water.

In the water, lying flat on my board while paddling out, felt good because now all the weight was off my spine. But I had made one fatal mistake. In my haste to get out in the water, I had failed to apply wax to the back part of my board. In the surfer's world, wax is more valuable than gold because it keeps you from slipping on your board.

While standing up on the first wave that I paddled for, my rear foot slid off the back of the board as I did the splits. I experienced intense pain as I heard a popping sound. At that very moment I knew I was in trouble, that I had made one of the biggest mistakes of my life.

The next day my right leg was numb and painful down to the toes. Because of my medical training, I was pretty sure that I had ruptured a disc in the lower part of my spine. It was time to see our neurosurgeon at the Air Force Regional Medical Center, Dr. Roberto Masferrer.

After Dr. Masferrer examined me, I was admitted to the hospital where the myelogram confirmed the presence of a large ruptured disc. My worst fears were true; it was decided that I would need surgery. This is where my story began.

After my surgery, the pain and numbness down my leg was greatly diminished. What a relief! But the pain in my back was excruciating. My back now had a huge hole in it. There was a gap between the rear portions of the two vertebrae where Dr. Masferrer had to cut away the bone to get to the ruptured disc. I thought the removed portions of bone would be rewired back in place. I was wrong. They were thrown in the garbage can and muscle was sewn together to cover the hole. I realized then that what Dr. Masferrer said was true. My back was indeed broken!

Upon release from the hospital, I was instructed not to drive or climb any stairs for one month. Two days later, I was driving my car and got locked out of my office at the hospital, so I had to use the stairs.

At home I had a pair of hanging boots that I used to stretch out my back. Following the axiom "physician heal thyself," I decided that I could give myself traction and get an upper body workout at the same time by hanging upside down while holding small dumbbell weights in my hands. Can you imagine the stupidity? Predictably, I never even made it that far!

Only three days out of the hospital, standing in the checkout line of our base's only department store with 30 pounds of dumbbell weights in my arms, I felt the left side of my back collapse.

As I stood there grimacing in pain, not speaking a word, a petite female store employee noticed my pale and clammy face and offered to take the weights off my hands. For the first time in my life, I, Mr. Macho, "superman extraordinaire," accepted help from a woman. As my male ego crumbled with my back, I noticed how grateful I was to be relieved of the physical burden of those weights.

When I reached home, however, the muscles in my back orchestrated a major spasmodic rebellion. They seized up violently, locked themselves into a deathgrip, knotted themselves into fist-sized lumps, and simply refused to budge. Laid out flat once again, this incident was a huge setback in my rehabilitation.

I was in so much pain that just going to the toilet was a major ordeal of the day, taking from 2-3 hours just to crawl down the hall on my hands and knees before returning back to my bed. Sitting on the john or taking a bath were impossibly excruciating, and I had to psych myself up for several hours in advance, anticipating this dreadful, yet necessary daily ritual.

Due to the proximity of the intestines to the spine, when my bowels moved they would set my back off in a wave of painful spasms. Thereafter I fasted on mango and carrot juice for two weeks to avoid any bowel activity whatsoever. Without any food in my intestines, I didn't move my bowels for the entire two-week period.

The Air Force gave me a choice. Return to work or face a medical board to go on disability with an early separation from the military.

Clearly, my back was in a bad way. This was despite the fact that I was now eating 10 mg Valiums and an ungodly number of other medications as if they were candy. These pills had no effect on the pain in my spine. All they did was make me feel stupid.

I thought about the Air Force offer and decided I didn't want to give in to the prospect of permanent disability. I knew if I had taken their money, that's precisely what would have happened. I've seen it too many times in my profession. "All that glitters is not gold," I reminded myself. To this day, I've never regretted my decision to decline disability.

Stubbornly, I forced myself back to work, refusing to cut short my service obligation. I donned a back brace and, swallowing pills by the handful, toughed out the next year, completing my tour of duty on schedule.

After my service was completed, like a wounded animal retreating to the safety of a cave to lick his wounds, I sought refuge in a quiet place. I needed a break from the world, so I journeyed to India to stay at a yoga institute. It was a very quiet place located in the remote highlands in the western part of the country. I had no car and no telephone and for the next seven months, instead of taking care of other people as I had been trained to do as a doctor, I concentrated on my own healing.

I decided to throw away my pain pills and face the pain head-on. After nearly a year and a half of dependency, this was a big step for me. Now I felt naked and vulnerable to my pain. It was frightening! But I was stuck in a hole and I wanted out. This was the obvious first step that had to be taken.

Without medications, the pain overwhelmed me, and I plunged into a deep, dark cavern of hopelessness and despair. Anybody who doesn't think that pain can drive a person to the depths of depression and despondency, to the point of contemplating suicide, has never experienced true pain. It is pure hell, nothing less! Nothing can demoralize your spirits like steady, consistent, unrelenting, chronic pain!

At the institution where I was staying, I followed a regimen that consisted of various stretching, breathing and relaxation exercises, reading inspirational books to keep my spirits up, and a simple diet that was free of toxins and highly refined, processed foods. I devoted myself exclusively to this program, and scheduled all of my daily activities around the healing of my spine.

All was not easy. During this period I had to deal with the tremendous physical, mental, and emotional exhaustion that the pain was causing. Every day, awakening to more pain after having worked so hard the day before, was demoralizing. My spirits were at an all-time low.

I was still in the process of trying to understand my pain and not be terrified of it, but my pain carried a huge psychological advantage over me of having completely intimidated me for almost 15 years. In other words, it was well-established in my psyche and could not be easily shaken.

During this period, I read all the experts' books on back pain and was not getting the answers I wanted so I threw them away and surrendered to the guidance of my own intuition and inner spirit. Because I was basically charting unexplored territory, I decided to trust my instincts and proceed from a very fundamental level.

I knew I had a body, and I believed that if I could learn to listen to it, it would guide me in the right direction. All I had to do was pay attention and work with the pain, accepting it as the voice of my body. My intuition told me that if I honored my body and was patient, the healing process would occur on its own.

According to the experts, I did everything wrong. I bent my body forward when I shouldn't have, and I knelt down in the wrong fashion. But I didn't care what the experts said because I was moving with more awareness than ever before and I was learning to listen to my body in a way that I knew was good for me. As I became acquainted with my body's wisdom, I began to hope that my personal suffering would soon come to an end.

After two months, I took a personal inventory. While I wasn't getting worse, clearly I wasn't getting any better and that was discouraging. Perhaps my expectation of a speedy recovery was unrealistic. I decided to get out my mental magnifying glass to measure my progress in micrometers instead of inches. In spite of my hard work, improvement was elusive. Depression and suicidal thoughts intermittently renewed their onslaught, and many times I felt like quitting.

After several months of floundering and experimenting, however, I began to notice small changes in my body that let me know I was on the right track. These were the first clear signs that the healing process was underway. With this encouragement, I continued on the course that I had set.

I found out later that the seeds of healing are sewn during such plateau phases where no apparent progress is being made. It is important not to get discouraged at such times, but rather to be patient.

One of the more helpful elements of my healing program while in India consisted of going to a large, flat rock in the middle of a secluded rice field and standing in the hot sun every afternoon for two hours at a time. With the heat searing down on my bare back, I would place my feet at different angles, practicing the simple art of standing. I stood in various positions, bending my knees, shifting the weight from one foot to the other as I changed the direction in which my feet were pointed, ever mindful of how these changes impacted the muscles of my back. I became acutely aware of the connection between my feet and back, and how I had not paid enough attention to this important anatomical relationship before. When I got tired of standing or when the pain became too intense, I would lie down with my back directly against the surface of the rock and let the radiating heat penetrate deep into the muscles of my back. Over a seven-month period, this large, flat slab of stone became my hospital and healing sanctuary.

I kept a journal by my side to document my insights and discoveries. I called it my Pain Journal. Proceeding this way, I found my body to be a huge storehouse of wisdom. Pain, I discovered, was one of the ways my body communicated this wisdom to me. I also discovered that painful memories were somehow stored in my body in the form of muscle tension, and that this pain could be released once I could relax and release the tension in my body.

As I stretched and moved my back, I began to see that I could no longer keep running away from my pain. I was committed to this journey; there was no turning back at this point. I was willing to face whatever pain I discovered in my life, wherever I found it.

Then, I began to understand that my physical pain, powerful as it was, was just the tip of the iceberg. A much deeper emotional and spiritual pain had been buried in my soul and suppressed for years. My physical pain was making me aware of my emotional and mental pain. As I worked with my body, I found myself reflecting on painful issues in my life, from incidents of my early childhood, up through the present day.

And I gained another valuable insight through this process. I had never learned to stand up for myself; I had avoided confrontation and interpersonal conflict at all costs. Learning to stand up physically required a corresponding commitment to stand up for myself mentally and emotionally, to take a stand on who I was and what I believed in. Did I have the courage to defend my principles and say no to others when necessary? If not, I would have to learn. It was amazing to discover that these deep, emotional principles could somehow express themselves in my body.

Through the help of my body, the deep layers of pain in my life were coming to the surface of my conscious awareness where I could confront the pain, understand it, and then release it. As I did, my body began to heal, so I knew I was heading in the right direction. I decided to follow the pain in my body. It was really as simple as that.

When I returned to the United States, I enrolled in a two-year training program in guided imagery, sometimes called visualization. I learned how the mind can heal through the skillful application of imagination. As I practiced what I learned, my back continued to improve.

I read John Bradshaw's books on the family and the need to heal childhood wounds. I enrolled in a week-long intensive course that dealt with this topic while I explored the relationship of my physical pain to deeper, unresolved emotional issues within my own family.

I was also assisted by many healers, including chiropractors, acupuncturists, osteopaths, massage therapists, yoga teachers, nutritionists, herbalists, and a host of others, some highly conventional, others quite unorthodox. Almost all of these healers helped me in one way or another, adding a new piece to the puzzle I was assembling on my way to reclaiming my wholeness.

The intimate relationship I discovered between my mind and body during this healing process was fascinating; I had no idea just how closely they were connected before I went through this ordeal. My pain was showing me how responsive my back was to my thoughts, particularly those that dealt with concern, worry, or fear. Such thoughts immediately made me feel a twinge or tightening of the muscles in my back and made me realize that they were causing tension in my body.

Positive thoughts wouldn't disturb my back in the least. They would actually relax it. I discovered that my thoughts could influence the health of my back, and that if I listened to my back, it would help me identify healthy, constructive thoughts that would not create tension or stress in my life.

I learned to consult my back at every possible opportunity. I would check with it before making important decisions. If something didn't make my back feel good, I would avoid it. In this way I allowed my back to influence my choices, and modify my lifestyle. As a result, my lifestyle is healthier today than ever before and so is my back. It proves that by listening to your body, you can enjoy a healthy, happy life.

Over the course of time, as I slowly climbed the psychological and physical mountain of pain, I began to sense a deeper mental and emotional purification taking shape. My body felt healthier, lighter, freer, more relaxed, and more flexible. It wasn't long before the pain was no longer in control of my life, even though it wasn't completely gone.

I now see that my back pain was a catalyst for a profound personal transformation in my life.

I am grateful for the understanding that my back pain brought me. It made me a better person and a more compassionate doctor. Without going through the pain, I never would have made the changes that were so necessary for my growth and evolution. I now see how pain is a blessing in disguise.

While pain descends upon your life initially as an unwelcome visitor, if you have the courage to study its deeper lessons, it will be a consummate instructor. Because pain has guided me into the spiritual fabric of my soul, the source of all healing, I can now offer you a way out of your pain.

CHAPTER TWO

Your Mind, Your Body, and Back Pain

YOUR MIND AND YOUR BACK are deeply and powerfully connected. To begin the healing process and to discover the real cause of your back pain, you need to understand this critical relationship.

First, and most important, you need to know that virtually all back pain begins with problems in the muscles. When your back muscles are tight, tense, weak, or out of balance, with the slightest provocation, like "the straw that broke the camel's back," you can easily suffer an injury, strain, or spasm, and intense back pain. I have seen this happen to people while they were sneezing, coughing, bending down to pick up a coin, or turning around to talk to a friend.

Of course, when there has been a more serious injury such as in a car accident or a fall, other structures of the back may be damaged. But it will still be the muscles that are the greatest source of your pain because they are directly connected to the nerves that transmit pain messages to your brain.

In the overwhelming majority of cases, problems in the back are created or made worse by stress or tension in the mind. When you are tense for a period of time, your muscles contract and they become more and more tight, stiff, and painful. You may not even be aware that you are mentally tense or under stress, but just as the hairs on the back of a cat stand up when it is agitated, your back muscles automatically tighten-up under stress. If you have had an injury, your back cannot possibly heal when the muscles are tense. In the absence of an injury, with tense muscles in your spine, your back is just an accident waiting to happen. As a rigid tree in a strong wind will snap, a stiff and tense back can go out in an instant. Tense muscles are much more susceptible to strain, spasm, injury, and, ultimately, pain.

Even if you have been told by your doctor that your back problem is the result of degenerating disc disease, bone spurs, spinal arthritis, a pinched nerve, scoliosis, or some other condition, remember that all of these conditions started with problems in the muscles of your back. When you restore the health of your back muscles, these conditions will be reversed, and you will, ultimately, be free of your pain.

By becoming aware of the critical role your mind and your back muscles play in the health of your spine, and by following the Back To Life Program presented in this book, you can heal your pain and strengthen your back no matter how long you have been incapacitated or how debilitating your pain might be.

Before you can begin to heal your back, however, you must understand how it works and how it fits into the greater scheme of your body's overall design and function.

How Your Back Works

Your spine* is one of the most important, sophisticated, and complex structures in your body. Almost every movement you make in some way affects your spine; that's how central your spine is to your overall good health.

---

* Please note that the terms back and spine are used interchangeably in this book. For all practical purposes, they refer to the same structure. Also, because the overwhelming majority of back problems occur in the lower spine, when I speak about the back or spine, I am referring to this area unless I state otherwise.

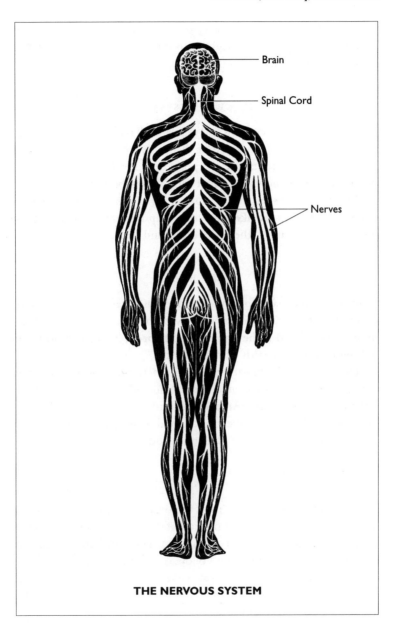

THE NERVOUS SYSTEM

The following structures and systems are critical to the proper functioning of the spine. Let's begin with the nervous system, the master system of the body.

THE NERVOUS SYSTEM

The nervous system controls and regulates all the other systems in the body. Its domain is so far-reaching that every single hair on your body has a nerve going to it; even the pores on your skin have nerves going to them. The nerves are what cause "goosebumps."

The nervous system can be thought of as the electrical system of your body. It looks just like a tree turned upside down, with a root (the brain), a central trunk (the spinal cord), and branches (the nerves).

THE BRAIN

The brain is the master organ of the nervous system. This makes it the most important organ in the body. **Even though the brain is usually not considered to be a part of your back, it exerts a powerful influence on the health of your back.**

The brain can be likened to a high-energy electrical transformer where impulses are generated and conducted throughout the body via the nervous system. An average adult brain weighs only three pounds but utilizes 20 percent of the body's oxygen supply. When an injury happens to the brain, the entire body can be affected.

THE SPINAL CORD

The spinal cord is one of the most important structures in your body. It can be thought of as a continuation of the brain, serving as the main electrical conduit of the nervous system. The spinal cord consists of long nerve tracts encased in a hollow, bony chamber formed by the vertebrae of the spine. This delicate cord-like structure runs from your neck down to the beginning of your lower back, serving as the body's main informational highway.

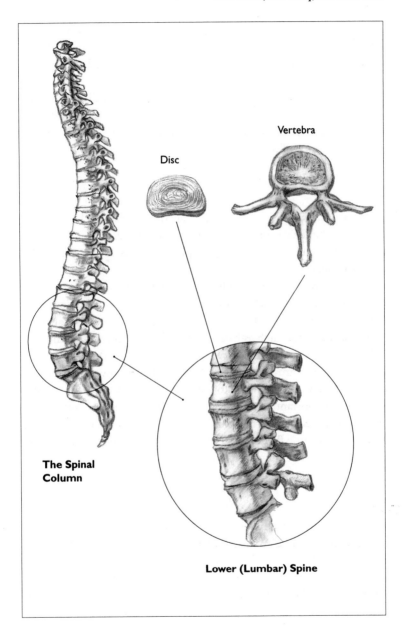

Disc

Vertebra

**The Spinal
Column**

Lower (Lumbar) Spine

The spinal cord is a vital link in brain-body communications. It relays messages between the brain and such vital organs as the heart, the blood vessels, the lungs, the kidneys, the intestines, and all the muscles in your body.

When an injury to the spinal cord happens, it is usually quite serious. Paralysis can result, affecting the legs, or both the arms and legs, depending on what level of the cord is damaged. We all know how tragic these kinds of injuries can be.

THE SPINAL COLUMN

The more than 30 bones of the spine, called vertebrae, stacked one on top of the other like a column, are known collectively as the spinal column. One of the main jobs of the spinal column is to protect and house the delicate and important spinal cord.

Another job of the spinal column is to help support the weight of the head, keeping the head and the brain in a level position while you're standing or walking. This is critical to the brain's processing of all vital sensory information such as balance, eyesight, hearing, and smell.

Nature has created several curves in the normal, healthy architecture of the spinal column. These curves have subtle yet powerful mechanical benefits and are essential to the health and well being of your spine. Most important among these are the concave curves in the neck and lower spine. These curves are technically referred to as *lordosis*. When they become flattened due to poor posture and unhealthy back muscles, serious back problems can occur.

THE DISCS

In between the vertebrae are marvelous natural shock absorbers known as discs. These circular, flattened structures are covered with a tough, fibrous lining and filled with fluid. They act just like the bushings in the shock absorbers of your car, cushioning the ride and making it smooth.

The function of the discs is to help absorb shocks to the spinal column

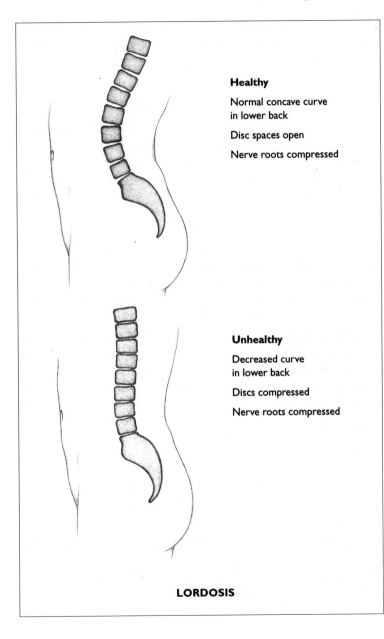

Healthy

Normal concave curve
in lower back

Disc spaces open

Nerve roots compressed

Unhealthy

Decreased curve
in lower back

Discs compressed

Nerve roots compressed

LORDOSIS

and facilitate the many movements of the spine as it bends forward and arches backward, as it leans from side to side, and while it twists in either direction.

SPINAL LIGAMENTS

The spinal ligaments are strong and flexible strands of elastic, fibrous tissue that look a lot like rubber bands. They come in a variety of lengths and widths, and help to support and buttress the vertebrae while protecting the spinal column against jarring and sudden, heavy blows.

SPINAL MUSCLES

There are literally thousands of muscles in the back that move and support the spine. They come in all shapes and sizes. There are long, thick muscles that run the entire length of your back, connecting the neck and head to the lower spine and pelvis. There are hundreds of smaller muscles, some less than an inch long, that connect adjacent segments of neighboring vertebrae. Another group of delicate spinal muscles attaches the vertebrae to ribs, so that even your breathing affects your spine as your ribs expand with each breath you take in.

What is truly remarkable about the muscles of your back is that tall, short, wide, thin, small, or delicate, they are all connected and choreographed to move as a harmonious unit with the most amazing grace and precision imaginable.

Your Back's Health Depends on the Health of Its Muscles

More than any other structure, including the bones, discs, and ligaments, it is the muscles of your back that determine the health of your spine. Keeping your back muscles strong, flexible, and properly balanced is the key to getting rid of your back pain.

An important job of the back muscles is to issue the first warnings

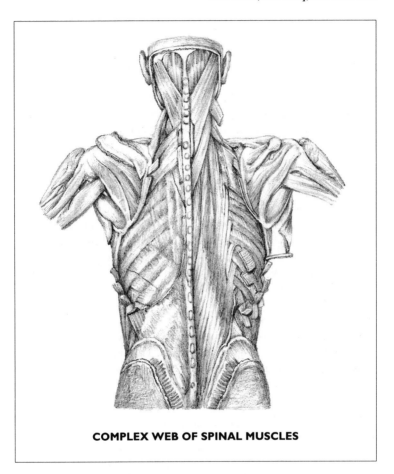

COMPLEX WEB OF SPINAL MUSCLES

—in the form of pain—when the health of your back is in jeopardy. Because of this, the bulk of the pain receptors in your back are located in the muscles. Almost all back pain has its origins in the muscles for this reason. When there is a problem in your back, it can almost always be traced to the muscles.

Two other critical functions of the back muscles are protecting the delicate spinal cord and aligning the vertebrae of the spinal column.

Your Muscles at Work

Understanding how the muscles in your body work will help you understand the muscles in your back. All muscles, including those in your spine, exhibit the following qualities and characteristics:

MUSCLE CONTRACTION

When the brain sends an electrical impulse to a muscle through the nerves, the muscle fibers contract. More electrical impulses, or greater intensity of stimulation, increases the force of contraction. When a muscle contracts, the bones to which it is attached will move. This is how movement in your body occurs.

MUSCLE STRENGTH

When muscles are contracted repeatedly, they can grow in size, especially if they are properly nourished. The larger the muscle grows, the stronger it gets. It is then capable of performing more work. This is known as muscle strength.

MUSCLE TONE

Even when a muscle is resting, there is still microscopic movement among its fibers, and therefore, contraction. This quality is known as the tone of the muscle, sometimes referred to as resting tension.

Tension or tone exists because of continuous nerve firing. The nerve keeps the muscle active and alive by firing at a low level of intensity, stimulating the muscle even when the muscle is not actively contracting. By being in this state of readiness, the muscle can spring into action more efficiently when it is needed.

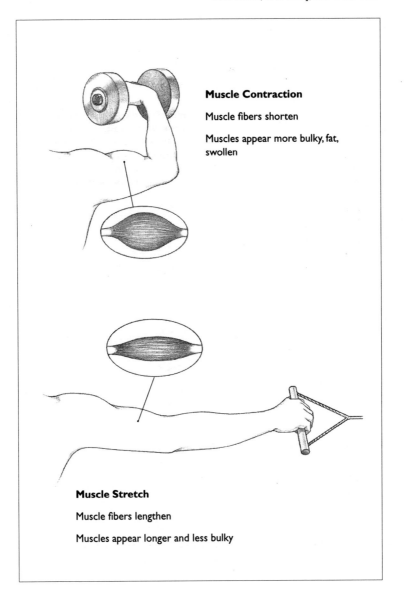

Muscle Contraction

Muscle fibers shorten

Muscles appear more bulky, fat, swollen

Muscle Stretch

Muscle fibers lengthen

Muscles appear longer and less bulky

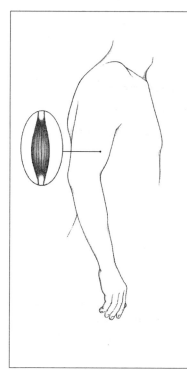

Muscle Tone

This defines the condition of the muscle while at rest. Increased muscle tone results from regular strengthening, but it can also occur in muscles that are tight and stiff from emotional or mental tension.

If the nerve to the muscle is injured, the muscle withers and dies and becomes paralyzed, as I mentioned earlier. It can't live without its electrical supply from the nerves.

Tension or tone increases in the muscle when the intensity or frequency of nerve firing increases. Therefore, increased activity in the nervous system can cause an increase in the tension or tone of the muscles.

MUSCLE STRETCH

Muscles are dynamic and basically elastic in nature; they can stretch when they are pulled. When muscles are stretched over time, they elongate and become looser and more flexible. With continued stretching, they can actually grow in length.

MUSCLE FLEXIBILITY

When muscles are stretched repeatedly, they become more flexible. This usually increases the range of motion of the joint across which they are attached. When muscles are tight and stiff, on the other hand, movement is restricted.

MUSCLE BALANCE

Every muscle in your body is balanced by an equal and opposite muscle. Muscles are paired to work in a complementary fashion to help synchronize the movement that occurs when they contract. These pairs of opposing muscles are known as antagonistic or complementary muscles.

Imbalance occurs when one of the muscles in a pair is either too weak, too strong, or too tight or tense. This causes unequal pulling of the muscles. Muscle imbalance can cause wear and tear on the joints, leading to chronic conditions like arthritis or other diseases. Healthy joints require healthy and balanced complementary pairs of muscles to facilitate smooth and efficient movement.

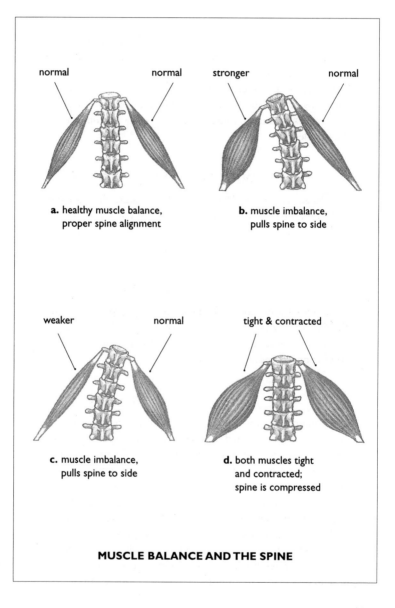

normal   normal

a. healthy muscle balance,
proper spine alignment

stronger   normal

b. muscle imbalance,
pulls spine to side

weaker   normal

c. muscle imbalance,
pulls spine to side

tight & contracted

d. both muscles tight
and contracted;
spine is compressed

MUSCLE BALANCE AND THE SPINE

THE SPINAL MUSCLES PROTECT
YOUR SPINAL CORD

The numerous and powerful spinal muscles safeguard the health of the spinal cord. The back muscles are the most sensitive muscles in your body for this reason. When there is a threat to the spinal cord, the supersensitive spinal muscles go into spasm and lock themselves in a strong, tight grip that is typically 10-20 times more painful than any other muscle spasm in the body. This restricts movement of the spine and protects the spinal cord from the risk of injury. The pain serves a protective function; it is an important message from your body telling you not to move any further or you could jeopardize the health of your spinal cord.

THE SPINAL MUSCLES
KEEP YOUR BACK ERECT

Another important function of the spinal muscles is to keep the back in alignment at all times. The muscles of the back help to maintain the spine's erect posture as you sit, stand, walk, run, and perform all the complex movements of the body. The muscles of the back and neck also support and move the head as it turns and rotates in a variety of positions.

Because the spine moves every time the body moves, the muscle mechanics of the back are extremely complex. When the muscles of the back are even slightly out of balance, they can throw the entire alignment of the spine out, resulting in severe pain.

Why You Need Healthy Back Muscles for Overall Good Health

The muscles of your spine not only determine the health of your back, they also play a critical role in the health of your entire body. In addition to performing the essential job of supporting your head and brain, they also participate in each and every movement you make.

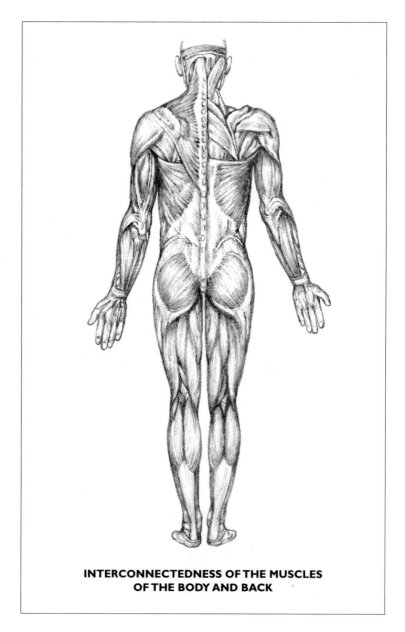

**INTERCONNECTEDNESS OF THE MUSCLES
OF THE BODY AND BACK**

This is because your back muscles are connected to almost every major muscle group in your body. You can think of your back as Grand Central Station, a crossroads at the center of your body through which all the other muscles must pass. The muscles of the arms, legs, and head all connect to the back at different levels. For example, the muscles of your upper back connect to your arms through the neck and shoulders, the muscles of the middle back connect to your chest and rib muscles, and the muscles of the lower back connect to your hips and legs. There is so much interconnectedness among these various muscles and the muscles of the back, that it is difficult to determine which muscles belong exclusively to the back.

Because so many muscles in the body are connected to the muscles of the spine, when any muscle is tight, tense, or spasming, a chain reaction of muscle spasms can start with potentially devastating consequences. It can throw your entire back out, resulting in severe and even incapacitating pain. People have thrown their backs out while throwing a ball, slipping on ice, stepping off of a curb, climbing stairs, leaning over a bench, reaching for a glass on a shelf in the kitchen, while sneezing or coughing, or as a result of all sorts of movements that may seem to have nothing at all to do with your back.

Because of these extensive muscular connections, when your spine is unhealthy, your whole body suffers. When your back is tight, tense, or undergoing muscle spasms, the nerves that come from the spinal cord become compressed, short-circuiting electricity to vital organs in the body. This impairs their function and damages their health. So it is critical to take care of your back muscles not only for the health of your back, but for your general health as well.

There are two muscle groups not located in the back that have particular influence on the health of your lower spine. They are the hamstrings and the abdominal muscles.

Your Spine and Hamstring Muscles

The hamstring muscles, located in the back of the thigh, connect to the bottom of the pelvic bone, which connects to the base of the spine. When the hamstring muscles are tight, they pull on the pelvic bone which pulls on the spine, flattening the normal lordotic curve in the lumbar area (see page 21). This puts all of the weight of the spine on the discs, creating an unstable condition which can cause extremely painful muscle spasms and throw the entire spine out of alignment.

In our modern way of life, where we do a lot of sitting, the hamstring muscles tend to be very tight. Many back problems can be relieved by taking regular breaks from sitting and stretching the hamstring muscles. It can really be that simple! The case of one of my patients, Stanley, clearly illustrates this point.

Stanley was a doctor in the community. He was also quite active in surfing, tennis, volleyball, and other sports. When his back went out, he came to me for relief. When I examined him, I found his hamstrings to be extremely tight and tense. I showed him how to stretch his hamstrings, which he did on a regular basis. Within a few days, his back pain was completely gone. While I also showed Stanley other stretches for his back, he continues to focus primarily on stretching his hamstrings, since for him this was the key. He's remained problem-free for over three years now.

Your Spine and Abdominal Muscles

The abdominal muscles provide important support for the lower back. Many experts consider the abdominal muscles to be an integral part of the spinal muscles; that's how important they are to the health of the spine.

When abdominal muscles are soft, flabby, and weak, they offer little or no support for the spine and place the spine at risk for injury or strain. When abdominal muscles are strengthened and toned, back problems often disappear.

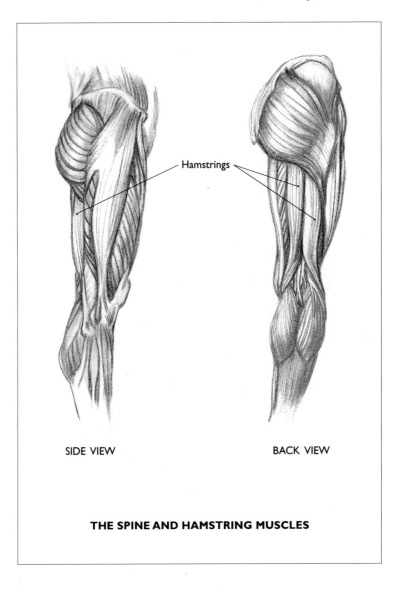

SIDE VIEW   BACK VIEW

THE SPINE AND HAMSTRING MUSCLES

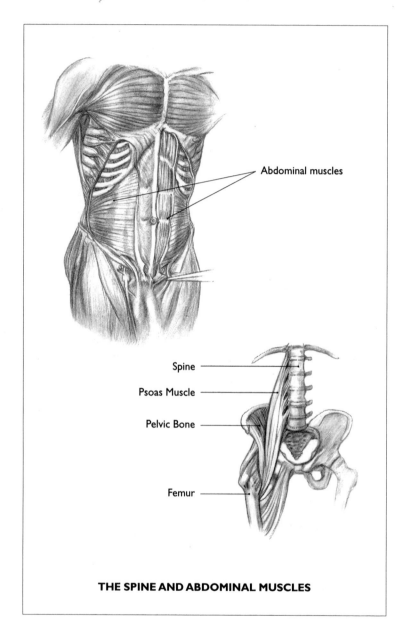

THE SPINE AND ABDOMINAL MUSCLES

The psoas muscles are powerful abdominal muscles that connect the bones in the upper thighs to the spine. They serve a very important role in stabilizing and supporting the spinal column. With a severe back strain or injury, pain in the back will often be accompanied by pain coming from both sides of the groin area. This pain is due to the psoas muscles, which lock into painful spasms to keep the spine from moving and possibly injuring the spinal cord.

Creating a Strong and Flexible Back

The muscles of your body are educable and open to change. Look at the bodies of professional body builders. They can make huge gains in strength, adding 100 lbs or more to the body's weight in pure muscle. They can sculpt their bodies by concentrating on the development of specific muscle groups in order to give them the kind of physique they want. Your muscles can be strengthened in the same way.

Your muscles can also be stretched and made very flexible. They can be trained to be highly loose, resilient, and elastic. Look at the yogis of India, sometimes called "rubbermen" or "pretzelmen," appearing to be double-jointed because of their amazing flexibility. By years of practicing regular stretching, they show us what is possible for our bodies.

Linda, a former back patient of mine, discovered the critical importance of stretching and strengthening her back muscles to get rid of back pain. Linda was a pastry chef at a nearby hotel and came into my clinic with excruciating low back pain that came on abruptly while she was bending down with a load of pastries. She had never experienced back pain like this before, and in her own words, it was worse than childbirth.

I could tell that Linda was out of shape. When I examined her spine, the muscles in her back were weak and stiff. I sent her for a course of physical therapy in which she learned specific strengthening and stretching exercises for her back. After just four weeks of stretching and strengthening her back, her pain was completely gone.

Even after surgery, you can create a strong and flexible back, no matter how many operations you've had. In my own case, where several pieces of bone and many muscles are missing from my back, I have been able to train what muscles I have left to the point where I can now teach yoga, lift weights, swim, jog, surf, hike with a heavy backpack, garden, and do many other activities better than most people who have never had a problem with their back. In fact, most people who see me engaged in these activities find it hard to believe that I ever had a problem with my back at all.

An interesting aside is that I have also gained almost one full inch in height after all the stretching I have done since my operation in which two discs were removed, a procedure that was supposed to make me shrink.

Now that you understand how the muscles of your back work, and how important it is to stretch and strengthen them, we can move on to a discussion of the powerful influence of your mind on your back.

How Your Mind Influences the Health of Your Back

Your thoughts are processed by your brain and transformed into powerful electrical impulses that travel through the nerves to all parts of your body, including the muscles of your back.

Your mind generates an average of 600–800 thoughts every minute. By simple arithmetic, that's an average of 42,000 thoughts per hour, 1,008,000 thoughts per day, 7,056,000 thoughts per week, or 366,912,000 thoughts per year! Since each one of these thoughts can generate electrical impulses that reach the muscles in your back, you can see what a powerful influence your mind has on your back.

Increased stress or tension in your mind translates into increased tension in the muscles of your back. When you are under stress, your tense and agitated mind produces a whirlwind of activity that creates an increasing number of negative thoughts. These thoughts are converted into numerous electrical impulses that directly contract the muscles in your back.

The Mind-Back Connection

To understand the critical relationship between your mind and your back, look at the following illustration to see the chain of events that occurs, beginning with your brain and ending in your back muscles. Here's how it happens:

1. Thoughts based on fear or worry excite or stimulate your nervous system.

2. Each negative thought generates tiny yet powerful electrical impulses that travel down your spinal cord and out through your nerves.

3. When these impulses reach your muscles, the muscles contract due to the electrical stimulation. With repeated stimulation, such as during times of mental stress or anxiety, your muscles become tight, tense, and often painful.

4. Your back pain causes more fear, anxiety, and worry, resulting in more negative thoughts, which further stimulate the nervous system.

This cycle perpetuates itself and escalates in intensity until either the pain or the anxiety are intolerable. At this point, conventional medical care is usually sought. A more practical, safer, and economical alternative to this dilemma is the application of the Back to Life Program outlined in this book.

As you now know, when a muscle is stimulated by the electrical impulse in a nerve, the muscle contracts. This results in a shortening of the muscle, which causes it to tighten and become more tense. The greater the stimulus, the greater the muscular tension and force of contraction.

One patient of mine named Joan had tremendous pain from her back that travelled down her right leg. The pain got worse when she and her young child moved into a house where she had an incompatible roommate. She admitted to me how stressed she felt over this arrangement. She decided to find another place to live. The day she moved into her new place, she felt the leg pain disappear altogether.

Your Mind and Your Posture

One clear example of the mind-back connection is your posture. This is your body language, and it can provide useful information about your thoughts and feelings.

Because your back muscles are directly influenced by your mind, your thoughts and the activity of your brain and nervous system can, over time, direct your muscles to shape the alignment of the bones in the spinal column into a certain posture.

For example, a depressed person typically demonstrates a drooping, slouched posture, shoulders drawn down and forward, with a low hanging head. Depression is written all over his or her body. In contrast, someone who is happy and joyous will automatically hold their head high, their shoulders back, their spine erect, in a very energetic, uplifting type of posture.

The Lie Detector Test

The lie detector test has been making use of the relationship of the body and the mind for years. It is so reliable that it is often used as admissable evidence in many courtrooms across the country. In lie detector tests, electrodes are connected from a person's body to a polygraph machine that measures muscle tension. Muscle tension in the body increases when people lie.

When a person lies, or tries to cover up the truth, tension is created by the increased amount of mental effort required to cover up each lie. This usually leads to a succession of lies that must be told in order to make the story credible. Underneath this elaborate mental process is the fear and anxiety created by the possibility of the lies being discovered. This creates more tension.

Some people think they can beat the lie detector test because they have all the angles covered. However, as each mental impulse gets transmitted to the body, the overall increased physical tension, which shows up in the muscles that are being measured, is a direct reflection of the mental tension caused by the act of lying.

We can tell if a person is lying or telling the truth by consulting that person's body with a simple lie detector test. The truth is, when it comes to measuring what is going on in the mind, the body never lies.

A Final Word

In order to heal your back pain, you need to understand what is causing it. When you can understand that your mind and your back muscles are intimately involved with your pain, you will take a quantum leap toward greater healing.

Here's a quick review of the most important points to remember:

1. Healthy back muscles are your key to a healthy back. When your back muscles are strong and flexible, they are healthy.

2. The pain receptors in the spine are located predominantly in the muscles, and it is from the muscles that almost all back pain arises.

3. The nervous system is the informational link between your mind and body. The brain sends messages to your body and the muscles in your back through nerves which originate in the spinal cord, the most important structure in your back.

4. Your mind and back are intimately connected. Negative thoughts can create stress and tension in your body, which will affect your back adversely.

5. Tension in the mind is directly translated into muscle tension. Mental tension and stress produce increased stimulation from the brain

and nervous system, which causes your muscles to tighten-up and become tense. Increased muscle tension in the back sets the stage for back injury and pain.

6. Back pain, which in the overwhelming majority of cases comes from the muscles in the back, can be healed through the natural, non-invasive Back To Life Program presented in this book.

CHAPTER THREE

Moving Past Your Pain

*Pain is the body's way of getting us to listen and pay attention.
When we have learned the lesson, the body will heal itself.*

S. Radha
Indian Author

PAIN CAN BE PURE TORTURE, a living hell, especially when it lingers on and on for weeks, months, or even years. I know; I have been there. But pain is also a blessing in disguise. It is a potent and powerful message from your body that warrants your undivided attention and understanding. It is your ticket and pathway back to health, happiness, and life.

In this chapter, you're going to look at your pain more closely than ever before to understand its purpose, learn from it, and, ultimately, overcome the fear it creates. Your pain will no longer intimidate you, and you will be able to heal your back.

Why Pain Means Life

Back pain can be intense, excruciating, incapacitating, frightening, and demoralizing, and yet, oddly enough, pain means life. Let me explain.

When a nerve to one of your legs is cut, the muscles in that leg become paralyzed, and you lose all feeling, including the feeling of pain. It's as if the leg goes to sleep and dies. Without nerve signals stimulating your muscles, the chances of your leg healing are quite slim.

Pain, on the other hand, demonstrates that your nerves are alive and causing your tissues to be active. When that happens, the opportunity for your body to heal is also alive. The chances of your leg healing are favorable. So you see, pain is beneficial in this sense: it shows you that the part of your body that is painful is alive and that it can be healed. **When pain is present, there is always the hope and potential for healing because pain means life.** When you lose the ability to feel pain, you may feel better, but you lose all hope of bringing life back to that part of your body, and with it, the opportunity to heal.

Your Pain Is a Message from Your Body

Pain is the language of your body. It is a message from your body's infinite well of intelligence that something is wrong. It is a natural impulse arising from within your body that has a beneficial and protective purpose. It warns you not to move in a certain way so that a part of your body that has been injured can heal. It forces you to listen to your body.

When you first experience pain, you just want to get as far away from it as possible. You are probably frightened by your pain and want to run to the nearest doctor or pharmacy for the strongest pain medication you can find.

But if you block natural pain messages with drugs, you will not hear the language of your body. It's like snipping the wires to the fire alarm in your house to shut off the loud buzzing sound it is making. Meanwhile, your house could be burning down and you wouldn't know it.

You can also do further harm to your back if you artificially block the body's normal pain response with pain-killing drugs. You might place your back in a position that can cause further injury and you wouldn't know about it. You wouldn't even have a warning. This is exactly what happened to me the day I took some painkillers, went surfing because I felt no pain, and ruptured a disc in my lower back.

Your body has its own naturally-occurring pain control mechanisms and you can activate them with specific strategies and techniques involving both your mind and body. Taking artificial chemicals to suppress the body's natural messages can be dangerous and harmful.

YOUR BODY'S NATURAL PAIN-CONTROL MECHANISMS

Endorphins and encephalins are powerful chemicals of the nervous system that your body uses to regulate pain. They are naturally-occurring compounds that are more powerful than heroin or morphine in modifying the pain response. When pain no longer serves the best interests of the body, these chemicals somehow block the pain impulses travelling to the brain.

Exercise is known to stimulate the production of these chemicals, helping to reduce the level of pain you experience. Laughter is another activity that is known to stimulate the production of endorphins and encephalins, as well as deep relaxation and stress management techniques (See Chapters Four, Five, and Seven).

Pain Is Nature's Reset Button

Pain helps you to grow and change when you need to take better care of yourself. Without being nudged out of your comfort zone from time to time, you can be lulled into a state of complacency that can be harmful to your health. Because it can't be ignored, pain forces you to do things differently and look at your life from a completely new perspective. Pain is nature's way of getting you out of a harmful rut. In the words of Bernie Siegel, M.D., "Pain is nature's reset button."

When a machine is malfunctioning, all you have to do is press the reset button and the machine will start up again. Pain serves this same function for you. It forces you to change the way you think, feel, and act. In doing so, you can elevate your awareness and improve the quality of your life by learning new ways of being and living.

Pain: A Mind and Body Experience

Pain is as much in the mind as it is in the body. Here's how it happens:

Pain receptors are located throughout the body. When they are stimulated, they send a signal to the brain that an injury or other problem has occurred.

As you know, the majority of the pain receptors in the back are located in the muscle tissue. When a muscle is stretched beyond its capacity, when it is strained, overworked or injured, or when it is spasming and knotted due to tension and tightness, the pain receptors are activated to send impulses to the brain.

The brain registers the fact that there is pain and brings it to the consciousness of your mind. So the sensation of pain depends upon your mind's awareness of it.

"Phantom limb" is a phenomenon that illustrates the mind-body connection of pain. It occurs in people who have had amputations of their arms or legs. Years after they have lost a limb, they can continue to experience pain as if the limb still existed. How can this be?

It demonstrates that pain is more than just a physical experience. It is in the mind as much as it is in the body.

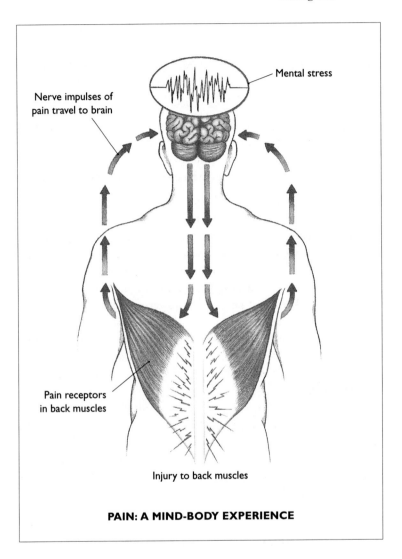

PAIN: A MIND-BODY EXPERIENCE

Why Muscle Pain in Your Back Is So Intense

Pain from a muscle strain in your back is typically 10-20 times more painful than a muscle strain in any other part of your body. This is because:

1. Your back muscles are designed to protect and defend the health of your spine and are supersensitive to pain for this reason.

2. The majority of the back's pain receptors are located in the muscles.

This exaggerated pain serves a function. The back muscles are part of your back's built-in "early warning system." They are programmed to sound an alarm whenever your spine is in trouble. Because the spine is so critical to your entire body's well-being, the alarm sounds an unusually loud warning. It can cause your back muscles to go into spasm, with excruciating pain that can linger for weeks, months, or even years.

However, when most people first experience incapacitating back pain, the last place they imagine the pain coming from is their muscles. They assume it is from a ruptured disc, a pinched nerve, or some other problem deep inside their spine. This compounds the problem because it creates more mental stress and tension, which in turn causes more back pain.

Your back condition will never improve until you learn to accept that your pain is coming from the muscles in your back, and then learn to work with your pain through stretching, strengthening, and relaxing your muscles, and managing your stress as outlined in the Back To Life Program (see Chapters Four and Five). This is the only way your back can heal.

Referred Pain from Your Back to Your Arms or Legs

Sometimes pain is felt a distance away from the location of an actual problem. This is called referred pain. Referred pain from the back

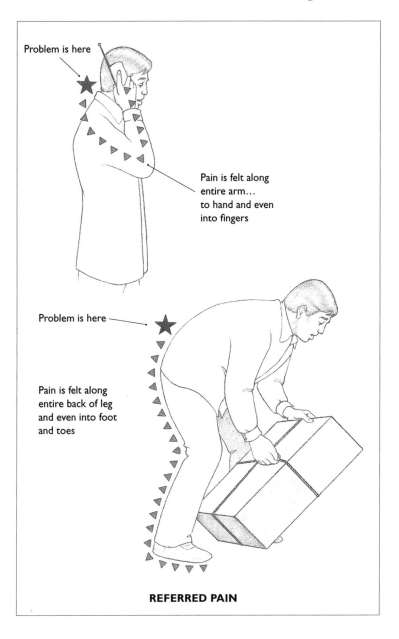

Problem is here

Pain is felt along entire arm... to hand and even into fingers

Problem is here

Pain is felt along entire back of leg and even into foot and toes

REFERRED PAIN

happens when a nerve root in the spine is compressed by a disc, due to a muscle spasm or imbalance. Pain can be felt along the entire length of the nerve, even though the problem is located at the root of the nerve where it exits from the spinal column.

When you have pain in your arm, even down to your hand and fingers, it could be referred pain from your neck. When you have pain down either leg, a condition known as sciatica, your pain could be referred from your lower spine. If this type of pain persists steadily for more than a month, it could be a problem that needs to be medically evaluated.

As you begin to apply the stretching and stress management practices described in Chapters Four and Six, and you have had referred pain in either your arms or legs, you may soon discover the pain diminishing. This is a favorable sign because it means that the nerve is becoming decompressed as the spine regains its normal alignment.

Muscle Imbalance and the One-Sided Nature of Back Pain

A study of Tour de France cyclists during an international competition revealed that across the board, the cyclists were favoring the use of the muscles on one side of their bodies by more than double the other side. This trend has been repeatedly observed in athletes from other sports as well.

The dominant side of your body tends to have stronger muscles because you use these muscles more. This means that the other side of your body is usually weaker. This commonly occurring muscle imbalance in the body leads to muscle imbalance in the back. Because of this imbalance, your back is at greater risk for being thrown out of alignment, and the resultant pain will often appear to be more on one side of your body than the other.

Strengthening the weak side of your back will help correct this imbalance (see Chapter Four).

Accepting Your Pain
While You're Healing

No matter where in your body you experience pain, it is important not to fight with it, hate it, or be angry with it. You'd be surprised to know how many people do this. Learn to accept that for now, there is pain in your life. That is the first step in the healing process.

I am not saying what so many other doctors say: "You'll just have to live with your pain." I don't believe you will have to live with your pain forever. I am proof of this. Pain should never be accepted as a permanent condition that you have to live with forever.

However, in order to move past your pain and get on with living the pain-free life you deserve, you first have to stop running from it, stop denying it, stop wasting your precious life energy being angry at it. First and foremost, be present with it, face to face, with the intention of learning to grow from it. To move past your pain, you must first accept it and make peace with it. The sooner, the better.

Climbing the Mountain of Pain:
Overcoming One Pain Parcel at a Time

In the beginning, when you decide to take the first steps towards overcoming your pain, the task can seem overwhelming. Your pain can feel too great. It is like setting out to climb a big mountain you have never climbed before. Looking up at the top, you are daunted by the thought of scaling such a lofty peak. The mountain seems so high, you don't know if you can do it.

One thing is sure, however. If you keep looking up at the summit, you will never reach the top. You will trip over your own feet and never make any progress. Progress is made by taking one step at a time, one day at a time, dividing your final, lofty goal up into small, workable goals, climbing only so high each day. As you achieve small goals, your confidence will build, and before you know it you will find yourself at the summit. This is how you climb any mountain.

Moving past the enormous mountain of pain in your back requires a psychological strategy just like this one. As you begin to work on those painful muscles in your back, keep the following points in mind:

1. Break up the total amount of your pain, no matter how great it is, into small workable units. Focus on one specific area of your back that is particularly troublesome to you.

2. Take the smallest unit of pain that you feel comfortable working with. Focus on it and don't look past it. This small parcel of pain is your current goal for progress.

3. Work with this parcel of pain using the techniques provided in the chapters that follow until it has disappeared completely. Don't set a time limit for how long this will take.

4. Once you have successfully overcome your current parcel of pain, you can move on to the next until, one by one, you have overcome each pain parcel and have completely moved past your pain. Before you know it, by applying this technique, you will have risen above the Mt. Everest of your pain. Slow but steady wins the race.

Breaking the Pain-Fear Cycle

One of the major obstacles to overcoming your pain is the fear that almost always accompanies it. When pain rears its ugly head, it can surprise and frighten you. Pain is almost always unexpected, and due to its intensity, it can literally send shock waves of fear down your spine. Pain can behave like a powerful monster. It can totally psych you out, incapacitate you, cripple you, and turn you into a psychological invalid, even if your body is still basically intact and healthy. What's worse, the fear that accompanies pain can increase the actual intensity of your pain.

How? It does so through the following mind-body connections between your brain, your nervous system, and your back:

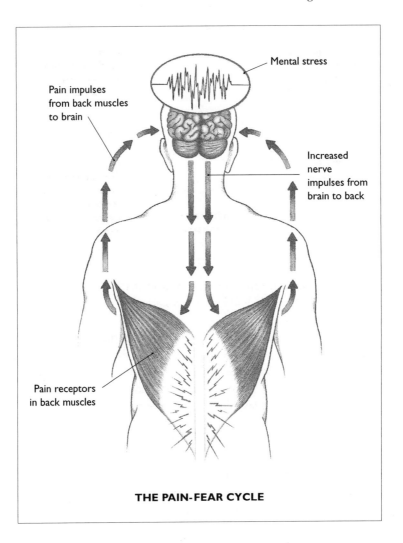

Mental stress

Pain impulses
from back muscles
to brain

Increased
nerve
impulses from
brain to back

Pain receptors
in back muscles

THE PAIN-FEAR CYCLE

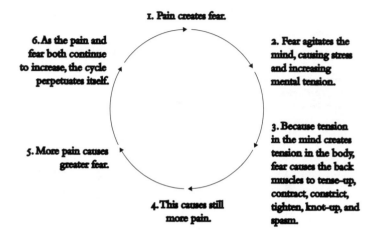

1. Pain creates fear.

2. Fear agitates the mind, causing stress and increasing mental tension.

3. Because tension in the mind creates tension in the body, fear causes the back muscles to tense-up, contract, constrict, tighten, knot-up, and spasm.

4. This causes still more pain.

5. More pain causes greater fear.

6. As the pain and fear both continue to increase, the cycle perpetuates itself.

This pain-fear cycle can be broken in two ways. If both are targeted simultaneously, the cycle will be broken faster, and your pain will go away more quickly.

One way to break the pain-fear cycle is by targeting the fear at the mental level with stress management techniques that help calm down and relax your mind. These techniques include relaxation, breathing, meditation, and visualization (see Chapter Six). When your mind is relaxed, your muscles relax. This reduces the pain in your body and diminishes your fear.

The cycle can also be broken at the physical level by directly stretching your muscles, (see Chapter Four), and by breathing and relaxation techniques (see Chapters Four and Six) that relax and release tension from the muscles in your back. This will diminish your pain. When your pain is diminished, your fear will subside.

Back Pain Is About
Slowing Down and Looking Within

Back pain always comes at the most inconvenient times. It hits right in the middle of your most frantic activity, when you are under the greatest stress, have a million-and-one things to do, and have important deadlines to meet.

Sometimes there is a delayed onset to back pain. It seems as if you make it through the most stressful times, and then it hits you hard and you end up flat on your back. In this scenario, it seems that the body musters a superhuman effort to make it through the hard times, but once the stress is over, it's as if all the accumulated stress catches up with you and now it's payback time, often with interest. In either scenario, back pain forces you to slow down.

At the Indianapolis 500, even the race leaders have to come in for pit stops to refuel, oil, lube, and service their machines at regular intervals. If not, they will be forced to take a pit stop due to some other reason. Since most people are so busy going, going, all day long, they don't take the time to listen to their bodies and find out why they need to keep going at such a frantic pace.

Back pain is nature's way of forcing you to take a mandatory pit stop, to rest, slow down, and take an inventory of yourself. It is an opportunity to listen to your body and heal yourself.

For those who don't accept this mandatory pit stop, the situation produces more stress. With the added stress comes added tension and pain. When you become completely incapacitated by the pain, your forward momentum will come to a grinding halt. Then you will be forced to not only slow down, but stop and face your pain.

Remember the story of the hare and the tortoise: Slow but steady wins the race. Life is like this. If you don't slow down and pace yourself, you'll never finish the race. (The stress management techniques in Chapter Six will teach you how to do this.)

Also remember that there is more to back pain than meets the eye. There are often deeper and subtler forces at work on your back than merely mechanical or physical ones. You can discover what these forces might be by quieting down your mind and looking within yourself. Try to go beyond the physical dimension of your pain to understand the deeper mental and emotional reasons for your back problems. One way to do this is to learn to listen to your pain (see also Chapters Four and Six).

Listening to Your Pain

When you are down and out with incapacitating back pain, it is the perfect time to practice the valuable technique of listening to your pain. Of course, even if your pain is only moderate you can still benefit. Listening to your pain is an art that is best practiced in conjunction with deep relaxation (see Chapter Six).

To learn to listen to your pain, follow these simple steps:

1. Allow yourself quiet, alone time to be with your own body. You will have to take time off from your busy life, go into a room, close the door, and take the phone off the hook so you won't be disturbed. Excuse yourself from your family duties, responsibilities, and obligations for at least 30-60 minutes a day, hopefully longer. The severity and urgency of your pain should justify your taking the time to engage in this extremely important healing activity.

2. Find a comfortable position, preferably lying down on your back with your knees or feet up, using pillows or blankets to support your spine.

3. Gently close your eyes, relax all the muscles in your body, and observe your body's natural breathing movements in the chest and abdomen. (See Chapter Six for instructions on relaxation and breathing.) Relax your mind.

4. With your body and mind relaxed, focus your awareness on your back pain and just observe your pain with a quiet, open mind.

5. Try to listen to your pain, not with your ears, but with your sixth sense or "inner knowingness," the intuitive part of you that knows what your pain means. Because your body has its own intrinsic wisdom, and since pain is the language of your body, see if you can understand what your pain is trying to tell you.

Your body is your greatest possession and it is important to get to know it better. Your body knows how to heal itself and when you are listening to your pain, you are learning to listen to your body. When you listen to your body, it will teach you how to heal.

Moving with Your Pain
After an Illness, Injury, or Operation

Imagine that your arm has been placed in a cast for one year. The cast extends from your upper arm to your wrist, completely immobilizing your elbow joint. Assume there was nothing wrong before the cast was placed on your arm. Now after one year the cast is removed. What will happen? How does your arm feel?

Your arm will be stiff. It will be so stiff, in fact, that it will be extremely painful to move at first. All the muscles will be tight, tense, and weak. Slowly, movement must be introduced so that the joint can regain its normal range of motion. Slowly, yet deliberately, the pain must be confronted as you gradually increase the range of motion for the joint. This will actually improve the health of the joint. It's the old adage of "move it or lose it." This is exactly what happens when people break their arms or legs, are put in casts, and after the cast is removed, must learn to regain normal use of their arms or legs.

When you begin to move your back after an injury or operation following an initial rest period, you can expect a certain amount of stiffness and pain due to lack of use. This is entirely normal. Don't let this stiffness or pain intimidate you from gently moving and stretching your back. To be safe, follow the guidelines in this chapter and

Chapters Four and Six, and you will see how quickly your back will recover and heal.

With surgical wounds and scars, it is important to remember that after the body has been operated on, tissues tend to shrink as they heal. The part of the body that was inflicted with the wound created by the surgeon's scalpel will be more tense, tight, and contracted as the wound continues to mend itself. This will cause a pulling sensation of pain in the center of the wound. This type of pain is a normal component of the healing process and should be expected.

After an initial rest period, it is important to go back into these painful areas to stretch the tissues (see instructions for stretching in Chapter Four). This will increase blood flow to the tissues and improve healing.

Overcoming Self-Destructive Behavior That Causes Pain

Before my back operation was about to begin, I asked my friend, Ben, who was a medical photographer at our hospital, if he would be willing to come into the operating room and take a picture of my back as it was being opened up by the surgeon. After he sent me a copy, I decided to frame it and hang it in my office as a teaching tool for my patients.

When I now show the picture of my bloody back operation to my patients, they wince in pain. I tell them that this is what people do to their bodies when they are self-destructive. When people are self-destructive, as I was, they are capable of this sort of behavior.

We all know the psychology of drug addiction, of smoking cigarettes, alcoholism, overeating, and practicing unsafe sex. These are all examples of self-destructive behavior. Having pain in your back can also be evidence of another form of self-destructive behavior. Much of this self-destructive behavior can be unconscious, that is, you may think you love yourself, but underneath, deep down inside where it really counts, you don't.

As Dr. Bernie Siegel said, "Sometimes my patients don't want to be healed. They are trying hard to die, so they come to me and get me to do their dirty work by slicing them open in an operation."

One patient in my clinic underwent 17 back operations! The record number of back operations on one person is, to my knowledge, 23. This is a clear example of self-destructive behavior, of masochism, even if it is unconscious. The surgeon is only the accomplice. When there is pain in the body, we usually go running to the doctor to fix us. If the pain is persistent and interferes with our ability to live a normal life, we will complain loud enough and long enough for the surgeon to find some reason why an operation is needed. If our pain doesn't go away with this operation, another operation will be recommended by either the surgeon, another doctor, or ourselves.

With each operation, the anatomy and architecture of the spine is altered and weakened, usually leading to more pain. Surgery can be lifesaving in many instances, and often, the pain subsides as the surgical wound heals. But if you return to old patterns of behavior, another straw will break the camel's back, and the same problems and pain will come right back.

No matter how many operations you have, sooner or later, if you want to truly heal, you will need to listen to your pain. A slow learner myself, I want to spare you the unnecessary pain and suffering that I went through. It could have been avoided had I taken the time to learn how to listen to my own body and honor the pain when I was first presented with this opportunity more than 20 years ago. The purpose of any illness or pain is to teach you how to be better than you were before, to grow, to heal, to learn to love yourself, and to discover a greater part of yourself. This requires an open mind, faith, and a lot of courage.

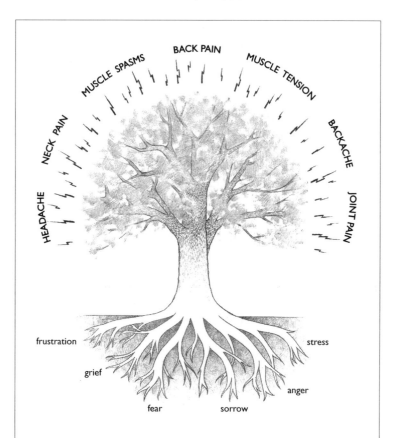

THE PAIN TREE

If you can think of pain as a tree, with roots, a trunk, branches, and leaves, then when you experience pain in your body, you are really experiencing only the leaves of the pain tree. In order to know and understand the roots of your pain, you must slow down the pace of your active life, quiet your mind, and learn to look within.

Overcoming the Emotional Roots of Your Pain

Chronic or ongoing pain almost always has emotional roots. When Dr. Bernie Siegel first shared this information with me, I didn't believe him. Now I realize that it is true. As Western medicine is just beginning to research and acknowledge the mind-body connection in health and healing, it is starting to recognize this very important principle. Sam's story is a good example of this.

Sam was an active person and hit the weight room on a regular basis to keep in shape. He also played baseball and surfed, in addition to doing his regular job.

Sam came to see me after his back first went out. He was in a lot of pain, but felt he only needed a prescription for some muscle relaxants and pain medication, a day or two of rest, and he'd be fine. He didn't mention it to me then, but on a later visit I discovered that his father was sick and near death in a hospital 6,000 miles away during this time.

Sam got better, but reappeared in my office within three months with the same problem. This time, he began to acknowledge that he was under a lot of stress and that he was upset because his father was dying. He was torn over having to go back to be with him.

Sam saw me several times after this, and his back improved when he did the stretching, but he couldn't see the value in the stress management techniques, or the connections between his emotions and his physical pain. He had always kept a tight lid on his emotions and intended to keep it that way.

At the one-year anniversary of Sam's father's passing, however, Sam's back went out again. He told me this time that since his last visit, he was much more aware of the tension he was holding in his body and in the muscles of his back over his anger, pain, and unresolved feelings he had for his father. He broke down and cried, something he hadn't done in over 20 years, acknowledging for the first time that the pain he was feeling in his back was in all likelihood a symptom of this much deeper emotional pain he was experiencing over the loss of his father.

How do you become aware of these painful emotions that are contributing to your physical pain? You do this by listening to your pain and practicing the other mind-body techniques that are prescribed in this book. Your pain is a teacher that can reveal all these things to you in time. Follow your pain, and it will show you the way to healing— not just the healing of your back, but to a much deeper healing of your entire being.

Whatever you feel, is registered in your body. Emotions generate powerful chemistry within your body, even if those emotions are repressed and you are completely unaware of their existence. Painful or traumatic emotions that get repressed at an early age get stored in the body and can create tension and stress.

Chronic pain is often a conditioned response to deep-seated feelings of guilt and self-blame. When we feel guilty, we unconsciously seek punishment, and punishment always brings pain.

Sharing Your Pain to Heal

Most of us have been taught to "grin and bear it," to keep our pain in and not let anyone else know about it. You don't want to burden others with your pain, so you learn to stuff it, keep a stiff upper lip, put on a happy face, and when asked how you are, reply, "Fine!" But people can see the pain on your face and in the way you carry your body anyway, so why not come out with it? I have learned that it is healthier to share your pain so you can release it and be healed.

In his work with cancer patients, Dr. Bernie Siegel learned that keeping pain in is unhealthy, eventually causes illness, and can accelerate your demise. Concealing your pain from others ultimately creates more pain in your life. When you genuinely share your pain, you heal.

Contrary to what you may have been taught as a child, sharing your pain takes courage. It is a sign of strength, not weakness. By sharing your pain, you are relieving your body of its burden, and in the process, you are giving permission to others to share their pain with you.

What kind of pain am I talking about sharing? All kinds. Especially the stuff that really hurts—the loss of a loved one, the pain of being lonely and isolated, of not being able to work because of your back pain. Just get it off your chest. You will feel more connected to yourself, your friends and family, and people in general, and you will feel the tension and pressure of your back pain lift. Sharing your emotional pain is physically healing.

A Final Word

Through my own suffering and subsequent healing, I realize that I have become a better person for having gone through the pain. My willingness to share my pain with others has helped me to grow, and the wisdom I have learned from my pain has turned out to be one of my greatest assets as a physician.

People who have survived and successfully overcome the pain and suffering of life-threatening disease almost unanimously report that when all is said and done, they are grateful for having endured their experience. They have learned how to love themselves and have discovered great inner strengths and gifts. Their illness and pain were wake-up calls to life.

I urge you, if you are suffering extreme pain, to stop running away from it as I did for so many years, and embrace it as a friend and teacher. If you do, you will be able to completely turn your life around and experience great joy.

Caution: While the overwhelming majority of all back pain comes from the muscles, in rare instances, pain can be caused by other problems. If you have experienced pain for over a month without relief, it is time to see your doctor and get your back evaluated. If nothing that requires immediate surgery is found by your doctor's evaluation, in all likelihood it will be safe to continue following the Back To Life Program.

CHAPTER FOUR

The Back To Life
Stretching Program

I N ORDER TO HEAL YOUR BACK and achieve a healthy spine, you must build up and nurture the muscles in your back in a way that will support and sustain proper posture and health. This is accomplished by systematic stretching and strengthening of not only the muscles in the back, but the other muscles in the body as well, since virtually all muscles in the body affect the back in one way or another.

In this chapter, I will take you through a series of stretching exercises that I call the Back To Life Stretching Program. These exercises will strengthen your muscles and eliminate back pain.

If your back is currently weak, tight, stiff, painful, or subject to getting thrown out of balance or alignment with the slightest provocation, you can reverse this situation by stretching and strengthening all the muscles in your body. This will make a tremendous difference in the health of your spine and the quality of your life.

Why Stretching and Strengthening
Your Back Is So Important

In our modern, sedentary society, our back muscles tend to become weak from lack of use. For instance, we sit while watching television, we sit when we go out to the movies, we sit when we eat, while we drive, at school, at the office, while at the computer, during meetings, on buses, in taxis, and in airplanes. With all this sitting, the back muscles just don't get enough exercise or movement. This makes them weak and stiff, prone to injury and strain.

In poorer countries where machines, furniture, and transportation are limited and people have to move their bodies much more than we do in order to live their daily lives, the prevalence of back problems is extremely low. "Move it or lose it" seems to be the general message when it comes to your back.

Stretching: A Vital Healing Activity for Your Back

Stretching is a powerful way to directly relieve pain from the muscles in your back. It develops flexibility of the spine and creates the conditions for your back to heal. It is probably the singular most important physical activity you can do to ensure that your back will be healthy for years to come. Stretching is also the most natural thing you can do, as every cat or dog will affirm. When you stretch, you release stored up tension in your muscles, releasing knots, tightness, spasms, and pain.

We have all seen football players warm up and do stretches before a big game. They do this because their coaches and trainers know that a relaxed and flexible body is much more resistant to injury than a stiff one. A flexible body is like a palm tree in a hurricane that can flex and bend without breaking due to its elastic and resilient nature. With all the crushing blows that football players receive today, stretching is the key to keeping their bodies loose and flexible, enabling them to play this rough sport while minimizing the risk of injury.

Stretching helps to heal injuries, as well as to prevent them. This is especially true for the back. Stretching is highly effective for chronic, degenerative conditions of the spine, or for conditions that have resulted from injuries and traumas that have been sustained over a long period of time. By eliminating the underlying tightness and stiffness in the body's musculature and surrounding tissues through stretching, the body can heal and become well again.

When you have any kind of problem in the spine, the highly sensitive back muscles tend to go into painful spasms. This is a protective mechanism of the body to keep you from moving your spine. At this time, the muscles of your back are in a state of constant contraction and tension, and the muscle tissue tends to become swollen and congested. Blood vessels become choked and constricted, and blood can't get into the muscle cells. The cells are then deprived of oxygen and they actually suffocate. This can cause more spasm and pain in the back. Toxins accumulate, resulting in inflammation along with more swelling and congestion. A vicious cycle at the cellular level of your back perpetuates itself.

Stretching helps relieve these painful spasms. When muscles are stretched, it's as if they can breathe again and return back to life. Stretching elongates and opens up muscle tissues. This helps to decongest the suffocated, tight, painful muscle tissues. Blood supply and oxygen delivery are improved when muscle tissues are stretched and toxins are eliminated.

When you stretch a specific muscle group, you are strengthening other muscles as well. Every opposing muscle in the body gets strengthened when you stretch its counterpart. It is impossible not to get stronger even if you are only concentrating on stretching.

Even if you are in severe pain, you can begin to stretch the muscles in your spine right now. Starting out slowly and gently, you can gradually increase the stretching as your back begins to loosen up and heal.

Caution: Pain is the body's unique way of telling you that something is wrong. In order to heal, you must learn to listen to your body. If pain occurs at any time while stretching, ease back until the pain goes away. If necessary, stop what you are doing and find a comfortable resting position. Also, if you have persistent pain going down either leg, a condition known as *sciatica*, avoid bending forward until the pain goes away. With acute back problems in general, avoid forward bending until your back feels much better. Stick to stretches that involve gentle backward bending.

Two Types of Muscle Pain

While we've established that the majority of back pain comes from muscle tissue, looking a little closer reveals that there can actually be two separate types of muscle pain. In each case, the sensation of pain will be slightly different. This information will help you as you begin to work directly with your pain through stretching.

Muscle pain can occur from 1) overstretching, a result of pulling too hard on a muscle, or from 2) overcontracting, a result of too great a workload, or too much stress and strain on the muscle that is being contracted. Both can cause a tearing of the muscle fibers and a painful knotting up or spasming of the muscle.

After your back has suffered a strain, injury, or operation, the predominant type of pain you will experience is from muscles that are tight, tense, knotted, spasming, and overworked or over contracted. However, you must also be aware of the muscle pain caused from overstretching because when you begin to stretch, you could easily stretch a muscle too far. This would only increase your pain and possibly cause more damage to your back.

Stretching into Your Pain

During the process of stretching, it is important to know how far to go. To stretch a normal, healthy muscle in a beneficial way, you need to stretch the muscle to the point just before any pain is felt. If you feel pain, you have stretched the muscle too far, and if you don't ease back on your stretch, you could tear and injure the muscle.

In the unique case of back pain, however, pain is already present in the muscles prior to their being stretched. Therefore, special instructions are warranted:

1. As you begin your stretching program, pay special attention to your pain.

2. When you stretch, notice how stretching and lengthening the muscle affects the pain.

3. If the pain becomes worse, the muscle is already overstretched. You need to back off of the stretch to the point before the pain starts and then hold the stretch there for as long as you are comfortable.

4. If the pain decreases, you are stretching the muscle in a beneficial way. Continue to stretch and lengthen the muscle as far as you are able to go before any pain of overstretching develops.

5. Try to stretch a muscle to its "edge," that zone of "pleasurable discomfort" that exists before the pain of overstretching develops.

Remember, pain forces you to grow and change. You must stretch into the pain to ultimately relieve it, but in a way that is intelligent and workable for you.

Preparing for Stretching

Keep the following points in mind as you prepare to embark on your individual stretching program:

+ Find a quiet place where you can be alone and undisturbed for 30-60 minutes. Shut the door if you need to.

+ Use props such as padding, pillows, blankets, rolled towels, belts, or other aids in any way you desire to help support your back or your arms and legs as you stretch. Be comfortable.

✦ Make sure the surface beneath you is comfortable. If it is too hard, use a mat or pad to cushion your body.

✦ Don't stretch on a full stomach. Allow 3-4 hours after a meal to do your stretching. For this reason, first thing in the morning before breakfast is a good time to stretch.

✦ Remove jewelry, watches, glasses, and shoes. Wear loose, comfortable, and unrestrictive clothing.

Before you begin the stretching exercises that follow, keep these additional points in mind:

1. **Stretch as far as you can without feeling pain.** If you don't stretch enough, the muscles will not become flexible and healthy. If you are feeling pain, however, you have gone too far. Ease back on your stretching and remain in the "pleasurable discomfort" zone, known as "the edge," that exists just before pain begins. A proper muscle stretch has a pleasurable pulling sensation.

2. **Don't overstretch.** If you push too far, you can tear and injure muscle fibers. Torn muscle tissue will contract and shorten as it heals, resulting in an even tighter and more tense muscle than you had before you started. This will cause more pain and make your back problem worse. If the pain in your back is so severe that you don't want to try any stretching at all, rest a day or two and then see how it feels before stretching again.

3. **If you are in excruciating pain, you can practice relaxation and start by slowly and gently stretching the muscles of your body that are not painful.** This will help to take the pressure off your back and lower the intensity of your back pain. Even a small improvement will help you to overcome the anxiety and depression that often accompanies back pain.

4. **Protect your back as you stretch by supporting it at all times.** Keep it in contact with the floor if you are lying down, or a wall if you are standing or sitting.

5. **If you are incapacitated by your back pain and cannot walk, start out with the stretches done in a lying down position.** You can start your stretching from the bed you are sleeping in. If you are sleeping on the floor, as is often the case with back pain patients, you can start your stretching from there.

6. **Do not bounce or jerk when you stretch.** Go slowly and steadily until you approach the pain, then stop and back off slightly. You will develop a feeling for what is the proper way to stretch because when done correctly, stretching feels good.

7. **Try to breathe slowly and deliberately when you stretch so that oxygen can enter into your body and nourish the muscle cells that are being stretched.** Try to become more aware of your body's natural impulses toward breathing as you bend your spine in different directions. You will notice that if you are forcing or straining while stretching, your breath will become shallow, rapid, and labored. Whenever possible, try to keep your breath slow, smooth, and easy. This will help you avoid forcing or straining your body.

8. **Don't force or strain or push through the pain.** If something hurts or doesn't feel right, don't do it. For whatever reasons, we all have a tendency to push beyond what's good for us. Honor your body and respect your pain. Don't fight with your pain. Don't grit your teeth and try to push through the pain. Don't ignore the pain. Also, try to avoid taking painkillers before stretching. They will numb the pain and mask the body's vital informational system. This could result in injury or further damage to your back.

9. **Whenever possible, stretch in the morning.** Even though your

body will be more stiff in the morning, you will have less fatigue at this time, your stomach will be empty, and after stretching your muscles and joints, your body will feel fresh and energized. This will have a beneficial effect on your mood and attitude, and start your day on a positive note. Your body will generally be more flexible in the afternoon and evening, but even though it may seem easier to stretch at these times, after a long day of working you may be more fatigued and less able to stick to an afternoon stretching regimen. If you do decide to stretch in the afternoon or evening, remember to stretch when your stomach is empty.

Relaxation and Stretching

It is very important to be relaxed as you stretch. Since this is a skill that must be learned like anything else, I'm including a technique that has been instrumental in the healing of my own back, as well as those of my patients. You can practice this technique whenever you want, as many times in the day as is needed. It is safe and effective, and although the technique appears quite simple, you will soon discover it to be one of the most powerful elements of healing your back that is offered in this book. Just follow these simple steps:

+ Lie down on your back, stomach, or side in a comfortable position. You may elevate your knees, hips, or legs using pillows, rolled towels, or blankets in any position that is comfortable for you.

+ Once you are comfortable, gently close your eyes and relax the muscles in your shoulders, arms, back, and legs.

+ Now bring your attention to your stomach and abdomen. Notice how they expand when your breath flows into your body. Notice how your stomach and abdomen gently contract when your breath flows out of your body.

✦ Let your attention move with the movement of the breath as it flows in and out of your body.

✦ Feel and observe the gentle up and down, rhythmic movement of your stomach and abdomen, noticing how your breath enters and exits your body of its own accord, without trying to control the rate or depth of the movement.

✦ Adopt the attitude of a passive observer. Just watch the flow of your breath as it moves in and out of your body, as if the breath were something different from yourself.

✦ Relax the muscles in your shoulders, back, legs, and entire body.

✦ Relax your mind and body as you continue to observe the movement of your breath as it flows in and out of your body.

✦ Let your mind and all the muscles in your body relax completely as your awareness moves with the movement of your breath, in and out, in and out, as if you were watching the waves in the ocean gently lapping up on the shore. Remain in this position for at least 5-10 minutes, and longer if you wish.

This relaxation technique can be done in a number of positions, either lying down on your back, stomach, or side. It relaxes the muscles of your back and entire body by calming your mind and your nervous system.

The Back To Life
Stretching Program

The following stretches are offered as a guide for you as you develop your own systematic stretching program. I have presented them in the general order of easiest first, but you must listen to your own body as you do each one. Here are a few additional tips before you begin:

1. On your first day, start with the stretches you can do and continue on until you feel you've reached your capacity for the day. Try to stick to a time limit, say 30-60 minutes, that you will be able to maintain on a daily basis. Instead of looking for the quick fix or the instant cure, try to develop a longer view. Healing takes time and is usually a gradual process, but with regular daily stretching, the time it will take your back to heal will be greatly shortened.

2. Allow yourself some flexibility (no pun intended) in following the program. Because everyone is unique, it is difficult to know in advance exactly what your body can tolerate. You may not be able to do all the stretches initially. In fact, very few people can. While the stretches are grouped starting with the easiest, you could skip over the ones you aren't able to do for now, and instead, focus on the ones you can do. You may, however, want to try a stretch first to see how it feels before deciding to skip it.

3. Feel the effects of each stretch on your body *as you stretch*, and *immediately following the completion of the stretch*. Don't try to make your body conform to the picture in the book. Instead, close your

eyes and feel your body from within, while allowing your breath to flow smoothly and slowly. The beauty of this program is that you don't have to be a perfectionist for it to work for you. Remember not to force or strain, stay relaxed, and try to be aware of your limitations. As your back heals, you'll see the limitations diminish.

4. With each new day, repeat the stretches you did the previous day, then add any new ones you may want to try, especially if you feel your back is up to it. As your back improves, you will want to progress from the easiest stretches in Phase I to the more difficult stretches. But proceed at your own pace. If you feel you overdid it the day before, or are tired, please take time to rest. Try to follow the stretches in the order presented in the book, but don't be too rigid. Listen to your body. Remember not to force or strain, and above all else, don't push yourself.

5. Don't get discouraged. Muscle knots, pain, tension, and spasms yield to persistent stretching. Muscles can get educated over time! They can stretch and elongate as your body becomes more flexible. And the more the muscles elongate, the more flexible your body and back will get. Your back will feel much better, lighter, and younger. A regular, daily stretching program will reward you tremendously. Be patient and you will see the results!

Note: The Back To Life Stretching Program described in this chapter, when done according to the guidelines provided, is entirely safe for the vast majority of back problems. If you are currently being treated for a special back problem, or if you have a question about your back, please consult your physician or a back specialist before undertaking this stretching regime.

A Few Words on Stretching

The stretches described in this chapter are in no way intended to be all-inclusive. They are a guide to help you get started if you've never stretched before. There are literally thousands of additional stretches available that can help your back. Once you learn to listen to your body, and especially your back, you might find yourself even inventing your own stretches. That's what I did and it has helped immensely.

People who stretch regularly have far fewer back problems than those who don't stretch at all. It's a simple fact of life. If the muscles in your body are tight and stiff, they are much more likely to be strained or injured.

If you follow the Back To Life Stretching Program, you will discover there is nothing more natural or safer than stretching. Nothing will feel as good either. When done properly, stretching is one of the most pleasant and beneficial experiences possible. When you listen to your body, it will tell you what it needs to heal, and it will tell you how it wants to be stretched.

Phase I Stretches

If you are in extreme pain or have never stretched before, this is the place to start. You can also start here if your back is tight, stiff, or in moderate or even severe discomfort. Stay with this group of stretches for at least one to two weeks or until you feel confident enough to add the stretches from the next phase. As you begin to add more stretches, remember to continue doing the earlier stretches that helped you.

KNEES-UP REST

This position takes the weight entirely off the spine. It relaxes the muscles in the knees, hips, and pelvis which further decreases the pressure on the spine. This is generally considered the most comfortable position when you are having severe low back pain. Many people even sleep in this position.

+ Lie down on your back so that your buttocks are up against the side of your bed or a chair.

+ Keeping your back flat on the floor, slowly place your legs on top of the bed or chair, keeping your knees bent at 90 degrees.

+ Relax your body, close your eyes, and focus on your breathing.

+ Stay in this position for as long as you like.

Note: As an alternative, you may place either pillows or folded blankets under your knees to achieve a similar effect.

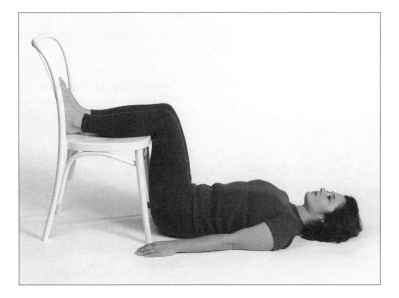

GLUTEAL SQUEEZES

If you are in severe pain and can't get off the floor or out of bed, do this stretching exercise. It strengthens the powerful gluteal muscles and helps to loosen and stretch the lower spine.

+ Lying on your back, slowly bring your knees up, keeping your feet on the floor. As an alternative, you can also relax your knees and keep your legs straight.

+ Gently squeeze the gluteal muscles in your buttocks as tight as you can and then slowly relax. Repeat this up to 100 times in the morning before getting out of bed, and in the evening upon retiring. Repeat as often as you like.

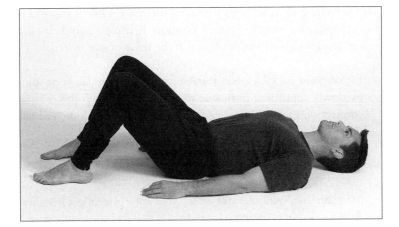

ALTERNATING BACK STRETCH

This stretching exercise helps to stretch the spine while it remains in a protected, non-weight-bearing position. It is especially helpful if you're in a lot of pain and can't get off the floor or out of bed.

+ Lie on your back in a comfortable position. Elongate your spine by slowly squirming from side to side as you stretch the muscles connecting each vertebra. Feel your spine growing long and tall. Breathe slowly and deeply.

+ Stretch both arms over your head, resting them on the floor.

+ Maintain this position as you stretch your left leg, feeling it lengthen. At the same time, stretch your right arm and feel your spine stretch and elongate. Stretch in this manner for a minute or so, then release.

+ Repeat this with the right leg and left arm, focusing on your breath as you feel your spine elongate.

+ As you alternately stretch the opposite sides of your body, feel your spine elongate.

+ Repeat up to 5 times per side. Focus on your spine and feel it elongating with each stretch.

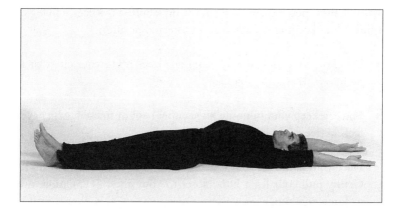

KNEE RAISES

Knee Raises stretch the muscles in the hips, buttocks, knees, and lower spine while keeping the spine in a protected position.

+ Lying on your back, slowly bring one knee up to your chest, or as high as feels comfortable.

+ You can keep your opposite knee either bent or straight, whichever feels better, as shown in the photographs.

+ Place your hands on your shins between your knee and your ankle. Gently pull your leg a little closer to your chest. Remember not to force or strain.

+ Breathe as you move, feeling the expansion of your chest and abdomen.

+ Feel the stretching in your hip joint, knee, and lower spine.

+ Repeat the same sequence with the opposite knee.

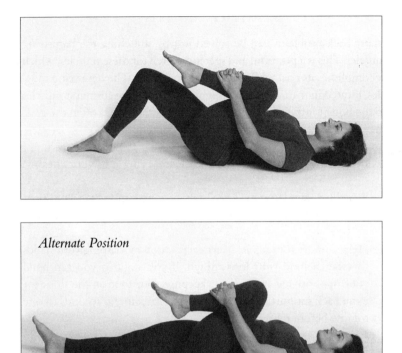

Alternate Position

STRAIGHT LEG RAISES

Many back problems can be solved just by stretching the hamstring muscles. This is a powerful and specific stretch for these muscles, which accomplishes its goal while protecting your back. The hamstring muscles, located in the back of the thighs, are among the strongest muscles in the body for their size. When they are tight, which is often the case, they can easily pull your back out of alignment.

+ Lying on your back, bend one knee and bring it to your chest.

+ Straighten your leg at the knee joint, holding it in a vertical position, as close to 90 degrees as you can without forcing or straining.

+ Help support your leg in a vertical position by clasping your hands together behind your lower thigh. If you want to you can bend your opposite leg at the knee, keeping your foot on the floor for extra back support. Try to hold this position for 30 seconds to one minute before releasing.

+ Feel the stretch in the back of your leg as you breathe in and out.

+ Rotate your foot at the ankle joint to enhance the quality of this stretch, noticing any tightness in your foot, ankle, lower legs, and the back of your thighs.

+ To release this stretch, slowly lower your leg to the floor, feeling the entire weight of your leg as you bring it down. If your back hurts when you do this, you can bend your leg at the knee and bring your foot to rest on the floor.

+ Repeat the same sequence with the opposite leg.

Note: It is essential to stretch the hamstrings, since almost everything you do favors their shortening and tightening, including sitting at a desk, driving a car, sitting and watching television, sitting on an airplane, jogging, riding a bicycle, and so on. Tight hamstrings put your spine at risk for further injury.

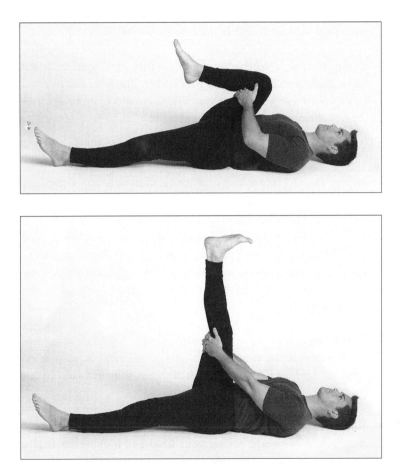

CAT–HORSE STRETCH

This stretches and loosens the muscles in the spine, increasing mobility and range of motion among the vertebrae while at the same time protecting the spine from the risk of further injury. Being on your hands and knees takes all the weight off your back, making it an ideal position from which to stretch and bring mobility back to the spine.

+ Slowly move from your stomach or your back onto your hands and knees. Make sure the weight of your body is distributed in an equal and comfortable way so that your arms, shoulders, hands, or knees are not straining due to excessive weight.

+ Adjust the width of your arms and knees so they are comfortable.

+ Notice how in this position all of the weight is taken off your spine, and that your spine can rest in this position.

+ As you breathe in, slowly arch your spine, particularly your lower spine, like a cat, lowering your head and relaxing all the muscles in your head and neck and shoulders as you stretch into the curvature of your spine, feeling any tightness, tension, or pain in any part of your back.

+ Maintain this position as you breathe slowly several times, allowing the muscles in your back to stretch and relax as your spine opens and releases. Allow the breath to move in and out of your body freely.

+ Slowly release the arch from your spine, and let it droop like an old swayback stable horse, raising your head and looking up as you form a concave curve in your spine.

✦ In this position, look up as you focus on your lower and middle spine, extending the buttocks upwards and breathing in and out in a relaxed manner. Feel the stretch in your neck, and upper and lower spine.

✦ You may go from the cat to the horse stretch up to 10 times on the first day, moving very gently and slowly as you do this. You can slowly build up to 25 times over several weeks, and you can repeat this number several times over the entire day if you feel the need to.

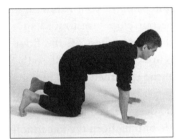

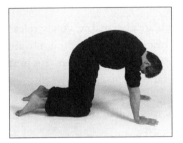
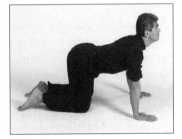

RESTING COBRA POSE

This stretch puts your spine in a position of extension, takes the weight off your spine, and opens the disc spaces so your spine can breathe. This helps to align your spine and restore proper posture.

+ Lie down on your stomach with your face turned to the side, your arms relaxed along the side of your body, and your legs relaxed.

+ Slowly bring your forehead to the floor, and bending your arms at the elbow, place the palms of your hands on the floor in line with your chest. Keep your elbows in toward your body. Slowly raise your head and then your chest off the floor as you move your elbows and hands underneath your chin so that the weight of your head is resting on the upturned palms of your hand.

+ Breathe slowly and deeply, relaxing the muscles in your lower spine as you feel a gentle pulling from the expansion and contraction of your stomach and abdomen.

+ Maintain this position as long as you are able before slowly releasing your arms and lowering your head back to the floor. Do this as often as you can. You can even read or watch TV from this position. Remember to breathe slowly and deeply.

+ When you are in extreme pain, try to spend as much time in this position as you can throughout the day.

+ If your pain is off to one side, try moving your hips away from the painful place in your back (see illustration).

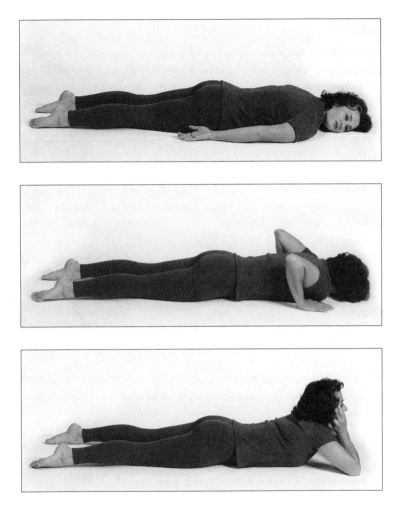

SERPENT POSE

This is an excellent stretch to improve the curvature of the spine. It stretches and elongates all of the back muscles, without the spine having to bear any weight. It also opens up the disc spaces between the vertebrae and decompresses the nerve roots.

+ Lie down on your stomach as you did in preparation for the Cobra Pose.

+ Keeping your palms in line with your chest as you did in the Cobra Pose, slowly extend your chin as you raise your head, neck, and chest off the floor.

+ Supporting the weight of your upper body with your arms and hands, slowly raise your chest and head as far off the floor as feels comfortable, breathing in and out as you do this.

+ Feel the expansion in your chest and the extension in your spine as you look up or focus your gaze straight ahead.

+ Breathe as you extend and relax your spine, relaxing the gluteal muscles in your buttocks as the muscles in your spine slowly elongate and stretch.

+ After 1 minute, or when you are ready, slowly come back in reverse order, eventually bringing your head back down to rest on the floor. Relax on your stomach with your eyes closed.

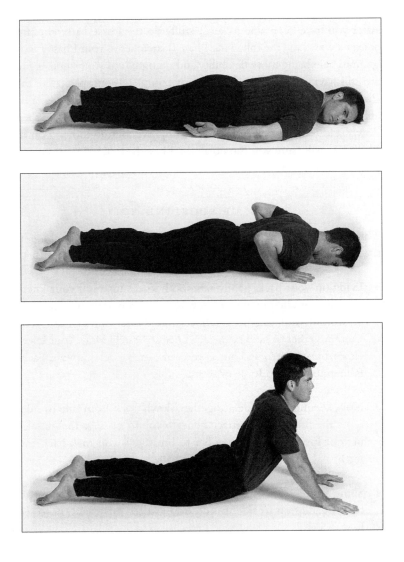

Phase II Stretches

After you have been able to successfully do the Phase I stretches for at least a week, add the following Phase II stretches to your Phase I program to help bring more flexibility and strength into your spine. If you are still having back pain, but are not completely incapacitated, the Phase II stretches will help take you to the next level. You may not be able to do all of these stretches initially. Do the ones you can, and then slowly add to your repertoire as you improve. Before moving on to Phase III, make sure you can do all the Phase II stretches without any pain or discomfort.

KNEES-UP ROCK AND ROLL

This is an excellent way to loosen and stretch your back first thing in the morning when you awaken, or after a long plane or car journey.

+ Lying on your back, gently raise both knees up. Hug your knees toward your chest by wrapping your arms around your bent knees or around your thighs, whichever feels better. Either clasp your hands together or hold onto each knee separately. Draw your knees closer, breathing in and out as you relax the muscles in your back. Remember not to force or strain.

+ Now, keeping your knees together, slowly rock from side to side, using the floor or the surface beneath you to massage the muscles in your lower back. Remember to breathe as you rock back and forth.

+ Some people like to rock from back to front and then front to back in addition to side to side. You can try this variation to see how it feels.

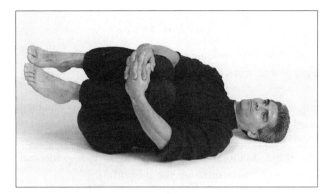

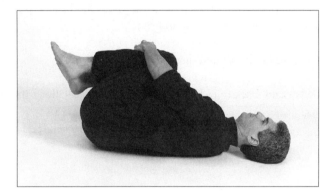

KNEE CIRCLES

This stretch tones the abdomen and strengthens and stretches the muscles of the lower spine, hips, and buttocks.

+ Lying on your back, gently lift your knees together and bring them toward your chest.

+ Move them slowly and deliberately in an ever-widening circle, keeping your lower spine on the ground.

+ Feel the connection between your stomach and back, hips, groin, and thighs as you breathe in and out.

+ After 5-10 circles, switch direction.

+ Slowly come back to rest, lowering your feet to the floor and then relax.

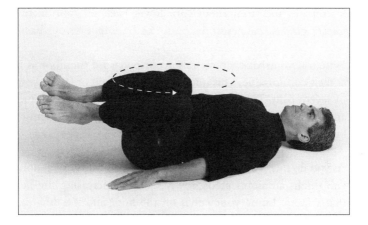

PELVIC THRUSTS

This stretches and strengthens your lower back in addition to the important gluteal muscles in the buttocks that support your back.

+ Lying on your back, slowly raise your pelvis off the floor as high as feels comfortable. This might only be an inch or two if you are in severe pain. Try to maintain this position for a few moments, and then slowly lower your pelvis to the floor. Remember to breathe as you move.

+ As you do this, feel how your lower back, hips, buttocks, abdomen, and thighs are connected. Slowly work at increasing the height that you are lifting your pelvis off the floor and the duration of maintaining at that height.

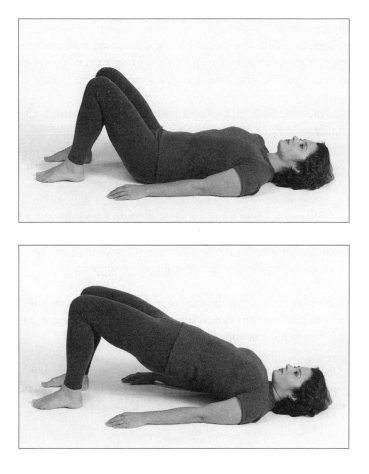

BENT-KNEE SUPINE TWIST

This stretch loosens the muscles in your spine via a gentle twisting motion. It is a very effective and safe twisting stretch for the entire spine and hips. Twisting is essential for overall spine flexibility.

+ Lie on your back in a relaxed position with your hands clasped under your head, elbows close to the floor.

+ Keeping your feet on the floor, slowly raise your knees, bringing your feet close to your buttocks.

+ Keeping your knees together, allow them to fall all the way to the floor on one side of your body or as far as they will go on their own. Let gravity do the work. Do not force or strain. You may want to put a pillow under your knees for support.

+ Turn your head in the direction opposite to where your knees are pointing. Close your eyes, relax, observe your breathing, and focus your awareness on your hips and spine.

+ After approximately 1 minute, or when you are ready, slowly bring your knees back to center, and then repeat this stretch on the opposite side of your body.

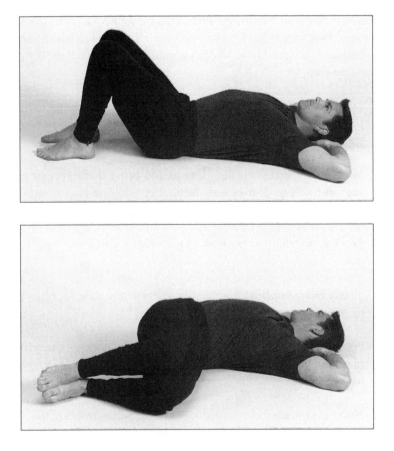

DOUBLE STRAIGHT LEG RAISES

This stretches your hamstrings while keeping your back protected. It is an excellent stretch for loosening your lower back and clearly defines the relationship between the muscles in your lower spine and the hamstring muscles.

+ Lying on your back, bend both your knees. Slowly bring them toward your chest, and clasp your hands together under the fold of your knees.

+ Now slowly straighten both legs, as you bring them upright to approximately 90 degrees with the floor or as high as you can without forcing or straining.

+ Feel the stretching in the back of both legs as you breathe in and out.

+ Slowly raise your head toward your knees as you slide your hands up your legs toward your feet.

+ Focus your awareness on the back of your legs, noticing the relationship between the muscles in your legs, lower spine, chest, and neck.

+ If you are unable to keep your legs straight while lowering them, you can bend at the knees and bring your feet down first.

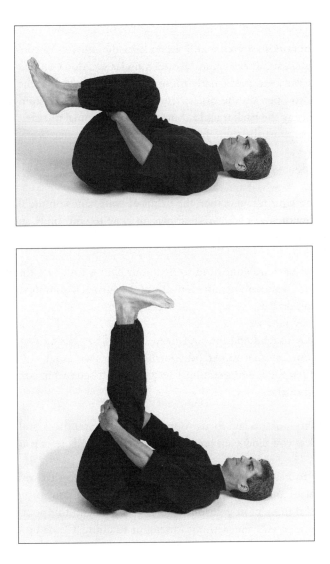

COBRA POSE

The Cobra Pose stretches and strengthens the muscles in your neck, upper back, and lower spine. It tones muscles you don't ordinarily use in your daily life, particularly those involved in extending the spine. It helps to open up the disc spaces while stretching and strengthening not only the back muscles, but also the abdominal muscles, which help to support the spine from the front.

✦ Lie down on your stomach as if you were relaxing.

✦ Bring your feet together, the palms of your hands on the floor, in line with your chest, your elbows up close to your body, and your forehead on the floor.

✦ Slowly extend your head so that your chin is touching the floor. Notice a stretching and elongation of your neck and upper spine as you do this.

✦ Slowly extend and lift your head off the floor, raising your chest as you continue to extend your head and neck as far as you can without forcing or straining. Feel a backward bending in your spine and breathe.

✦ Try to look up and focus your awareness on your neck and upper back as you allow your breath to move freely in and out of your body.

✦ Try to keep only light pressure on your palms so that your back muscles are doing the work in this stretch. Try also to relax the gluteal muscles in your buttocks as you maintain this position for as long as you can without forcing or straining. Come up only as high as is comfortable for you.

✦ Come back in reverse order, lowering your chest, then your chin, then your forehead to the floor. Turn your cheek to one side, close your eyes, observe the movement of your breath as it flows in and out of your body, and relax.

Note: As a variation, the Cobra Pose can be done with your hands clasped behind your back, and arms extended. See last photo for correct position.

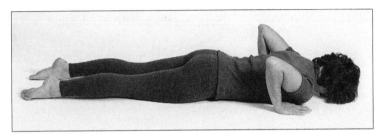

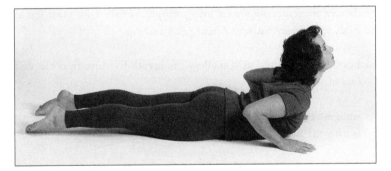

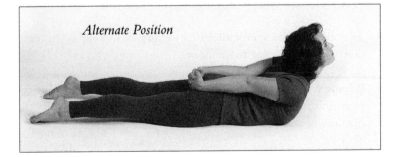

Alternate Position

HALF-LOCUST STRETCH

The Half-Locust Pose stretches and tones your lower spine by isolating the muscles of your back, working one side at a time. It also stretches and tones the muscles in your hips, buttocks, and thighs, which connect to your lower back. This is a very safe, effective, and powerful pose to help stretch and strengthen your back. It has been one of the key poses to strengthening and improving the health of my spine.

✦ Lie on the floor on your stomach keeping your feet and legs together.

✦ Slowly bring your chin to the floor.

✦ Stretch your left leg out behind you, pointing your toe like a ballet dancer, then, keeping your knee straight, slowly raise your leg as high as you can without forcing or straining.

✦ Look straight ahead as you allow the breath to move freely in and out of your body.

✦ Imagine that someone is pulling your leg upwards and backwards from your foot.

✦ Keep your body in a straight line as you focus your awareness on your hips, buttocks, and lower spine.

✦ After holding for approximately 1 minute, or as long as you can, slowly lower your leg to the floor.

✦ Repeat with the opposite leg. When you have finished, relax on your stomach with your eyes closed, cheek to the side, observing the flow of your breath.

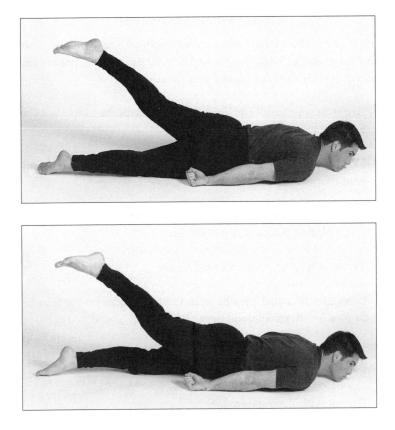

KNEELING HALF-LOCUST

This is an excellent stretch for your hips, and it strengthens and tones your lower spine. Some people find this variation a little easier and more enjoyable than the regular Half-Locust Pose.

+ Begin on your hands and knees as you did with the Horse and Cat Stretch (see page 86).

+ Slowly stretch one leg behind you as far as you are able, keeping your foot on the floor.

+ Keeping your knee straight, slowly raise your leg as high as you are able, pointing your toe as you do this.

+ Try to keep your body in a straight line.

+ Look straight ahead, breathe in and out, and focus on the muscles in your lower, middle, and upper spine.

+ After approximately 1 minute, or when you need to, slowly release the stretch.

+ Repeat with the opposite leg.

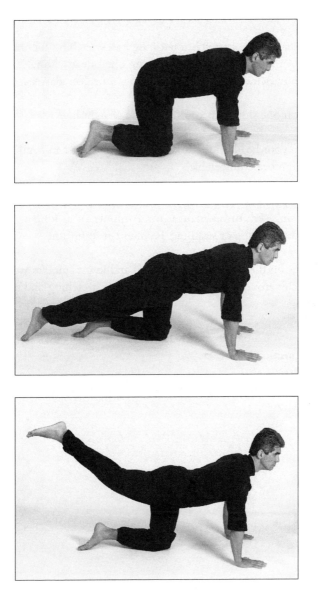

SIDE LEG RAISES

This is an excellent stretch for toning and stretching the muscles in your lower spine and hips. By isolating one side at a time, it helps to focus on muscles of the back that are often neglected, weak, and stiff.

✦ Lie on one side with your body in a straight line.

✦ Keep your head on the floor or rest it on your hand and elbow if this is more comfortable.

✦ Slowly raise your top leg as high as you can without forcing or straining. Try to maintain it for 1 minute or as long as you can without forcing or straining. Remember to breathe.

✦ Focus on the muscles in the lateral and lower spine as well as the muscles around the hip joint. Feel them stretching and strengthening.

✦ When you are ready, slowly lower your leg back down to the starting position.

✦ Roll over on your opposite side, and repeat this stretch with your opposite leg.

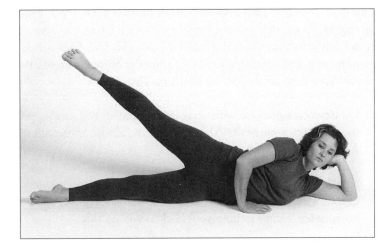

SIDE HALF-BOW POSE

This pose gives a gentle backward stretch to your spine which opens up the disc spaces between the vertebrae. It stretches and loosens the muscles in your lower back, hips, and shoulder blades which connect to your neck and upper back. This is a very convenient stretch that can be done even while you are watching TV.

+ Lie on your right side with your legs extended. You can support the weight of your head with your hand and elbow, or you can rest it on the floor.

+ Slowly bend your right knee and catch hold of your right ankle or foot with your right hand. Keep your elbow straight as you pull on your leg, gently arching your back as you do this.

+ Feel a gentle stretching in your back up through your shoulder blades as you use the muscles in your legs and arms to help elongate and extend your back muscles.

+ Slowly relax and return to the starting position.

+ Roll over and switch sides, repeating this stretch with the opposite leg and arm.

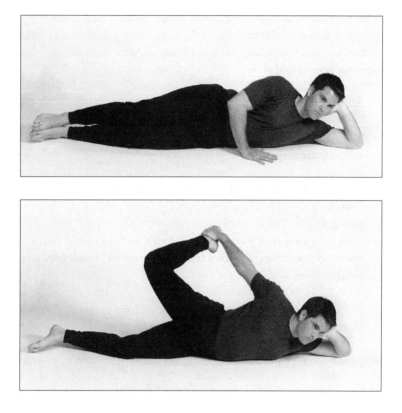

MOUNTAIN POSE

This stretches and strengthens your entire spine as well as your legs, feet, and shoulders. It strengthens the muscles in your legs and calves which support your back, and helps bring stability and balance to the nervous system and spine.

+ Stand with your feet together on a firm surface.

+ Slowly extend your arms and hands in front of you as you come up on your toes.

+ Bring your arms and hands over your head as you continue to stretch.

+ Feel the elongation in your spine as you breathe in and out, balancing on your toes, and stretching your arms and hands over your head.

+ Try to maintain this position for 30 seconds to 1 minute, focusing your gaze on one point in front of you.

+ Slowly come back and release the stretch.

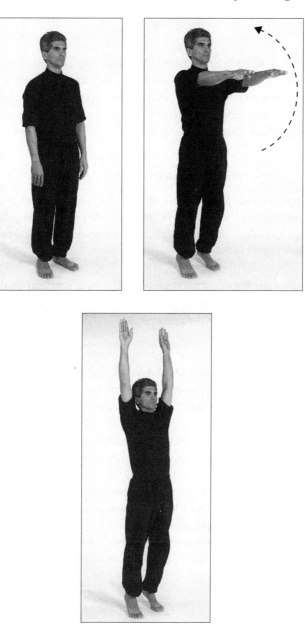

Phase III Stretches

These stretches are slightly more advanced and should not be attempted when you have severe back pain. They are, however, excellent stretches for your spine, and once you are over your initial trouble, if done regularly, they are your best insurance policy against any future problems with your back.

PELVIC POSE/JAPANESE SITTING POSE

This position completely takes the weight off your spine while stretching and opening the hips and pelvic bones that connect to your spine. It helps to realign the spine with a natural lordotic curve (see Chapter Two, page 21).

+ Place your knees on the floor beneath you as you lean on the back of a chair or sofa for support. Make sure your knees are on a soft and padded surface for this stretch.

+ Gently let the weight of your body shift back to your hips and buttocks. Slowly lower the weight of your body onto your knees, lower legs, and feet, going as far as feels comfortable for you. (This may take several weeks or even several months to do comfortably.)

+ You can place a pillow or folded blanket behind your knees in the beginning if you are experiencing discomfort on your knees.

+ Relax your body, sitting with your knees folded and your lower legs and feet tucked under your buttocks. Bring your shoulders back and sit with an erect spine.

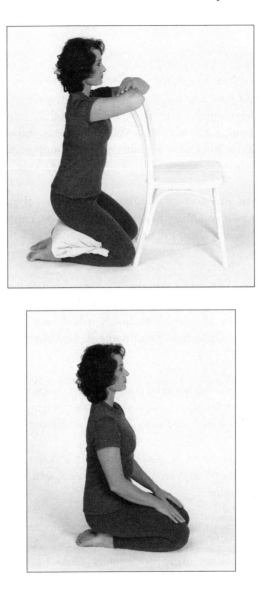

SQUATTING

This is an excellent stretch for your lower spine, while strengthening the muscles of your legs and hips which support your spine. It helps to open the lower spine while taking the weight off the spinal column. In the beginning, if the muscles in your hips, knees, and inner thighs are stiff, you can hold onto a railing or other support to help you maintain balance.

+ Stand with your feet in a comfortable position, about shoulder width apart. If you like, you can stand near a post, railing, desktop, or the back of a chair, and use your arms and hands to help support you.

+ Slowly bend your knees, keeping your spine straight, and allowing the weight of your upper body to come down on your knees and hips. Take care of your knees. If you have a knee problem, only come down as far as feels comfortable. Relax your spine as you do this.

+ Feel the relationship between your knees, your hips, and your lower spine as you relax your back and allow the weight of your upper body to stretch the muscles in your hips and lower back.

+ Let gravity do the work as you breathe in and out. Try to maintain this position for 30 seconds to 1 minute. Come back slowly in the reverse order.

Note: In poor countries where chairs and furniture are lacking, people tend to squat a lot. Because the incidence of back problems is so low in these countries, many back experts believe squatting is a large contributing factor.

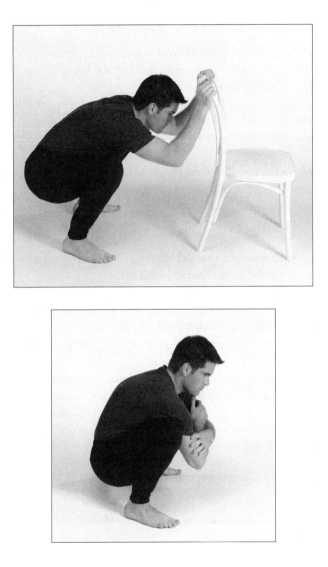

KNEELING–BACK ARCH

This stretch extends and gently twists the muscles in your entire spine. It strengthens and stretches muscles that run the length of your back, and helps to restore good posture.

+ Kneel on a padded surface so that you are "standing on your knees." Make sure your knees are comfortable and supported.

+ Slowly bring one arm straight up, away from your body until it is over your head. Continue to stretch it and bring it back all the way behind you until it rests on the back of your foot, your ankle, your lower leg, or wherever is comfortable for you.

+ Bring your opposite arm and hand up directly over your head and look up toward your outstretched hand.

+ Breathe into your belly as you arch and stretch your spine, extending and elongating it with every breath. Notice the relationship between your belly and your spine as you continue to breathe.

+ Feel the gentle twist and stretch in the muscles of your entire spine as you maintain this position for 30 seconds to 1 minute.

+ Slowly come back and repeat this stretch using the opposite arm and hand. When you are finished, relax.

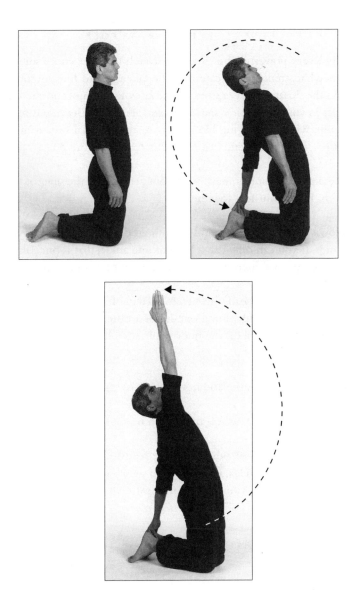

BOW POSE/HALF-BOW POSE

This is a very powerful and excellent stretch for your entire spine. It is somewhat strenuous, so care must be taken not to force, strain, or overdo the duration of the stretch. The Bow Pose tones and stretches muscles in your hips, spine, shoulders, and abdomen. Because it opens the spine while improving blood flow to the internal organs in the abdomen, it energizes and brings vitality to your entire body.

+ Lie down on your stomach with your arms along the sides of your body. Keep your feet together.

+ Slowly bend your knees and catch hold of your ankles with your hands. If you can only catch hold of one ankle, that is fine. In that case, keep your opposite hand stretched out in front of you.

+ Slowly raise your head, chest, feet, and legs off the floor at the same time. If you are only doing one leg at a time, you may also bring your arm and hand off the floor while stretching them in front of you.

+ Remember to breathe and not to force or strain!

+ Try to look up as you feel the stretch in your entire spine.

+ After 30 seconds, or when you are ready, slowly come back in reverse order and relax. If you need to switch legs, after your breath returns to normal, you can repeat this stretch with your other leg.

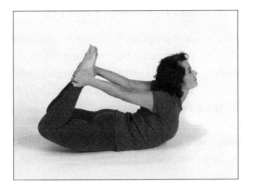

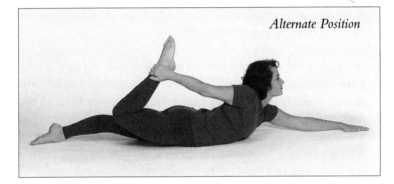

Alternate Position

HALF-SPINAL TWIST

The spine moves in six directions. Twisting to the right and left are two of these directions. Twisting helps to keep the spine supple and loose, and can release tension, tightness, knots, and spasms in muscles that are difficult to reach by other kinds of stretches. Twisting helps keep your spine truly flexible.

✦ Sit in a comfortable position with your legs extended in front of you. Try to keep your spine straight.

✦ Slowly bend your left knee and bring it toward your chest, but make sure it is not too close in. Check to see that your left foot only comes as far as your opposite knee.

✦ Bring your left arm and hand out in front of you and then slowly rotate your upper body and your head as you bring your left arm and hand all the way behind your back. Bring your hand to the floor with your fingers pointing away from your body.

✦ Sitting with your back erect, look over your shoulder as far behind you as you can, steadying yourself with your left arm and hand. Feel a twisting in your spine as you do this.

✦ Take your right arm and bring it across your knee as a lever to help you twist a little further. Only do this if it feels comfortable for you.

✦ Breathe and relax as you maintain this position for a minute or two. When you are done, slowly release the pose and repeat the same stretch with the opposite side of your body.

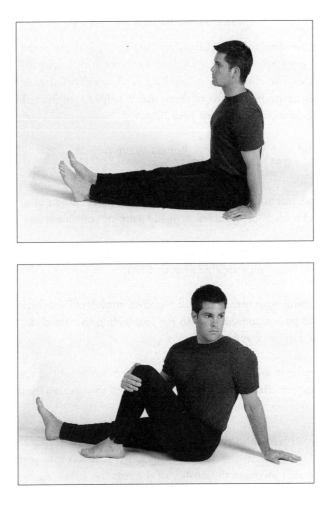

SIDE BENDING

Lateral bending to the right and left, like twisting to the right and left in the Half-Spinal Twist (see page 122), constitutes two of the six movements made by the spine. This is an excellent stretch for the muscles in the lateral part of the spine. It helps to improve the range of motion and flexibility of your back.

✦ Stand with your feet together on a firm surface.

✦ Keeping it more or less straight, slowly lift your arm up, with your hand reaching out to the side of your body. When your arm is level with your shoulder, turn the palm of your hand face-up.

✦ Continue to bring your arm up over your head until your upper arm is touching the side of your head.

✦ Keeping your arm and head together, stretch tall and then slowly bend your spine sideways to the left, feeling the stretch in the lateral part of your spine.

✦ Breathe in and out, relax, and try to keep the weight of your body evenly distributed over both of your feet, so you aren't putting all of your body's weight on one foot.

✦ As you remain in this position for 30 seconds to 1 minute, try to feel your breath expand your ribs when it enters into your body, so that it increases the quality of the stretch.

✦ Slowly come back and return to a relaxed standing position when you are done. Repeat this stretch with the opposite side.

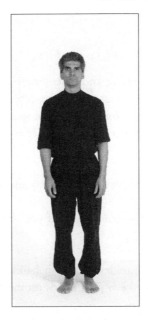

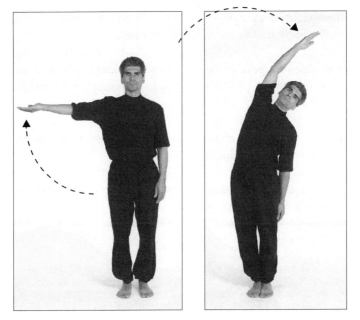

BRIDGE POSE

This is an excellent arching and extending stretch of the spine that strengthens and tones the muscles in your entire back. It stretches your shoulders and neck while opening the disc spaces in your back. While improving posture, this stretch increases energy and vitality in your entire body.

+ Lie on your back with your arms along the sides of your body.

+ Bring the heels of your feet toward your hips, keeping your feet on the floor.

+ Catch hold of your ankles with your hands if you are able. If you are not able to, just keep your hands on the floor.

+ Slowly raise your hips as high as you can, arching your spine. Allow the weight of your upper body to rest on your shoulders, upper back, the back of your neck, and your head.

+ For added support, bring your hands under your hips or lower back, using your elbows and arms to help support the weight of your body.

+ Breathe in and out and try to relax your spine in this position. Avoid forcing or straining.

+ After 30 seconds to 1 minute, or when you are ready, slowly lower your body to the floor and relax.

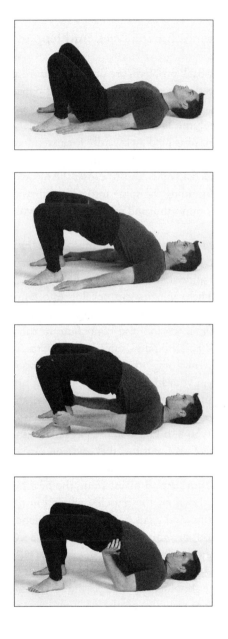

Stretches for the Neck and Upper Back

Neck and upper back problems are occurring more and more as people spend more time reading, writing, doing paperwork, and performing other tasks while sitting at computer terminals, office desks, behind the wheel in traffic, on airplanes, and while watching TV.

Because the head is held awkwardly for extended periods of time during these activities, the muscles in the neck and upper back can easily become strained. Over time, this causes the muscles to become stiff and tight while molding the spine into a bent-forward position. This contributes to poor posture and renders the spine vulnerable to injury and strain.

A common cause of strain to the muscles of the neck and upper back is whiplash. Whiplash results from violent thrusting forces applied to the neck and spine that occur during high speed auto collisions or "rear-enders." These injuries can develop into chronic tension and pain, and unless properly treated, are difficult to heal.

Stress and mental tension also contribute to the problems of the neck, upper back, and shoulders, since muscles in these areas are among the most prominent storage sites of stress in the body. When there is stress or tension in your life, it can invariably be found in the form of tight and tense muscles in your upper back, neck, and shoulders.

Consider a person who works at a computer terminal eight hours a day, has had a whiplash injury in the past, and is under considerable stress. Add all these elements together and you can see why neck and upper back problems are so common.

The key to restoring and maintaining the health of the neck and upper back is to focus on the muscles, which must be stretched and kept flexible, strong, and relaxed. Stress management techniques such as deep relaxation, breathing, and meditation (see Chapter Six) are also of paramount importance.

The neck muscles originate in the upper back and to some degree in the area of the shoulders. To stretch and loosen the muscles in the neck, you must not only stretch the neck muscles, but also the muscles in the shoulders and upper back, since they are all interconnected. The same holds true for the upper back. Focusing on stretches that treat these areas of your body as if they were all one, interconnected unit will promote maximum healing.

A Word on Referred Pain

Pain or numbness going down either arm, extending into the hands and fingers, indicates nerve compression, a condition usually originating in the neck area. If these symptoms increase while stretching, you are pushing too far in your stretch. Decreasing the intensity of your stretch should help alleviate the pain. Remember that any unexplained pain that persists for more than one month needs to be checked out by your doctor. (See also Chapter Three, page 46)

Shoulder-Opener Series

This series of stretches opens the shoulders, while stretching the muscles in the upper back and base of the neck.

HANDS BEHIND BACK

+ Stand with your feet apart, hands clasped behind your back.

+ Stretch your arms downward, keeping your elbows straight. Then, bring your outstretched arms away from your body by rolling your shoulders out and back.

+ Open your chest as you breathe in deeply, feeling the stretch in your shoulders, upper back, and the base of your neck.

+ Release this stretch after 30-60 seconds. Repeat 3-5 times, 2 or 3 times a day.

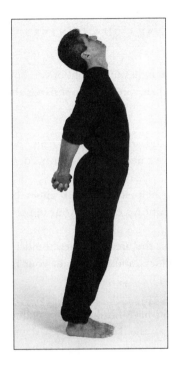

HANDS ON COUNTERTOP

✦ Place your arms straight out in front of you on a countertop or the back of a sofa or chair, spreading your hands about shoulder-width apart.

✦ Kneel down or stand, stretching your arms, shoulders, upper back, and the base of your neck. Relax your head.

✦ Allow gravity to help stretch your upper back and shoulders, putting a gentle concave curve in your upper back area.

✦ Feel the stretch in the area of your shoulder blades, middle and upper back, shoulders, and the base of your neck. Hold the pose for 30-60 seconds.

✦ Release when you have finished. Repeat this stretch as often as you can throughout the day.

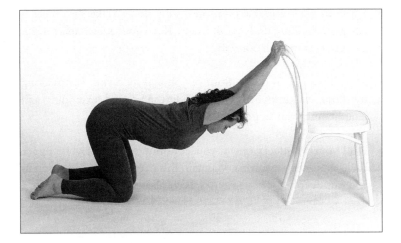

CHILD'S POSE

+ Kneel in a comfortable position on the floor. Make sure there is adequate padding under your knees. Keep your knees apart if this is more comfortable for you.

+ Stretch your arms out in front of you and slide your hands along the floor, walking your fingers along the ground, extending and lengthening your upper back as you stretch.

+ Roll your shoulders out as you continue to stretch your upper back, shoulders, and arms. Maintain this stretch while breathing in and out deeply for 2-5 minutes. Repeat a minimum of 3 times a day.

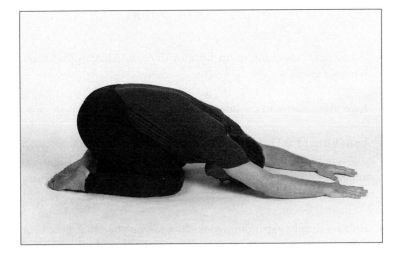

WALKING INTO DOORS

+ Stand in the opening of an interior door, one that is preferably standard width.

+ Extend your arms to the sides, placing your hands on the door jams.

+ Lean forward as far as you can without forcing or straining, making sure to keep your balance. Feel the stretch in your shoulders and upper back, rolling your shoulders out to stretch the area between your shoulder blades.

+ Breathe deeply, expanding your chest as you stretch. Adjust your feet forward or backward to increase or decrease the intensity of the stretch.

+ Hold this stretch for 30-60 seconds at a time. Repeat 3-5 times throughout the day.

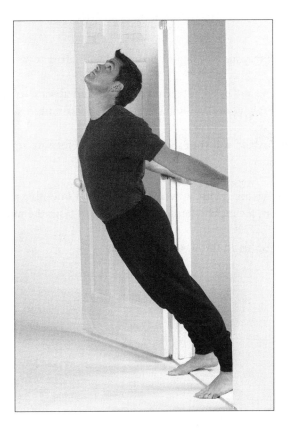

SHOULDER ROTATIONS

✦ Stand with your feet slightly apart and your arms at your sides.

✦ Breathe in and draw both shoulders back and upward toward your ears as high as you can without forcing or straining.

✦ As you exhale, roll your shoulders down and forward to the starting position.

✦ As you do this gentle movement slowly and smoothly, relax your shoulders, feeling the tension being released from the muscles.

✦ Repeat up to 10 times, 3-5 times a day.

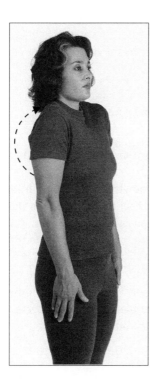 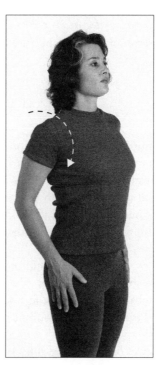

Neck Series

This series of stretches specifically targets the neck muscles.

BRAHMA MUDRA

+ Sit in a comfortable position with your shoulders relaxed.

+ Breathe in and out gently as you slowly bring your chin forward until it comes close to your chest. Feel the stretching in the back of your neck and try to look up toward your eyebrows. Maintain this position for 5-10 breaths.

+ Now slowly lift your chin and extend your head backward, focusing your gaze at the tip of your nose. Notice how the muscles in the back of your neck feel. Gently press your teeth together and feel the muscles in the front part of your neck.

+ Slowly bring your head back to level.

+ Slowly rotate your head as far as you can to the right without forcing or straining, looking over your shoulder as you do so.

+ Hold this position and breathe in and out, feeling the stretch in the muscles of your neck.

+ Now bring your head all the way around to the opposite side and repeat this stretch.

+ When you are finished, return to the starting position.

✦ This series of movements constitutes one round. Do 10 rounds 2-3 times a day, and see tremendous improvement in the health of your neck in 3-4 weeks.

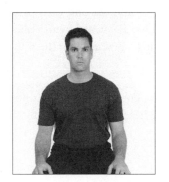

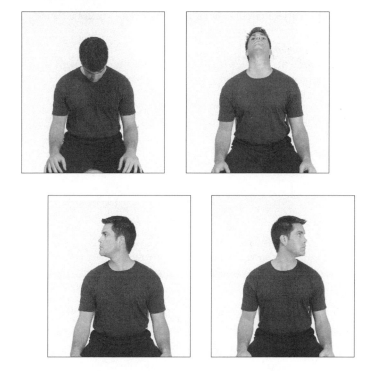

NECK ROTATIONS

✦ Slowly rotate your neck in a circular fashion, starting with small circles and gently widening the movement as you are comfortable. Breathe in and out as you move, noticing any tension in the muscles of your neck.

✦ Relax the muscles in your neck as you do this, releasing tension with every exhalation. Try to let your head hang limply without any strain on your neck muscles.

✦ Reverse direction after 1-2 minutes.

✦ Repeat these circular neck movements 3-5 times a day.

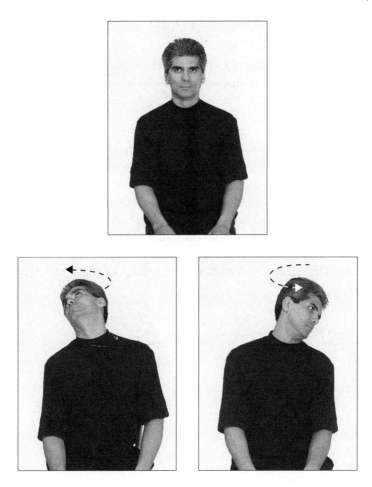

SUPPORTED NECK EXTENSIONS/ROTATIONS

✦ Lie down on your bed facing up with your head hanging over the side. Slide down so that you are able to let your head hang down as far as possible.

✦ Slowly rotate your head from side to side, breathing as you move, going only as far as the muscles in your neck permit. Be aware of any tension or pain in your neck muscles during these movements.

✦ As your neck begins to loosen, try to slide down so that a little more of your head lies off the edge of the bed. Do this for 2-5 minutes or longer if there is no discomfort.

Note: This can also be done in a seated position in a high-backed chair or sofa.

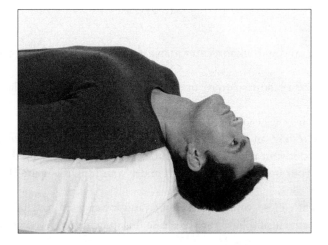

FISH POSE

+ Lie on your back in a comfortable position with your legs together.

+ Place a pillow sideways under your upper back and shoulders.

+ Arch your head and neck back so that the top of your head is gently resting on the floor and you can feel a stretching in the front part of your neck. Keeping your arms outstretched along the side of your body, tuck your hands under your hips, if you are able.

+ Gently close your mouth (upper and lower teeth touching) and breathe in and out slowly. Release this stretch after 30-60 seconds. Repeat 3 times a day.

+ To increase the intensity of this stretch, roll the pillow and place it lengthwise beneath your shoulder blades.

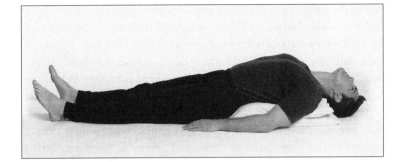

Stretching for a Healthy Posture

One of the purposes of stretching and strengthening the back is to help restore a healthy posture to the spine. A normal, healthy posture for the lower spine has been designed by nature in such a way as to possess a naturally occurring backwards curve, giving it a slight "sway-back" look. The technical term for this curve is *lordosis*. When we speak of the normal, healthy lower spine in terms of posture, we call it *lumbar lordosis* (See also Chapter Two, page 21).

By curving the lower spine backwards, nature in her wisdom knew that this would keep the body's center of gravity and weight distributed more on the rear and stronger parts of the vertebrae than on the forward portions where the discs are also located. Since the forward parts of the vertebrae are mostly filled with air and are less dense and therefore not as strong as the rear parts, they are incapable of bearing large amounts of weight for a prolonged period.

Stretching and Yoga

The stretches included in this chapter are all derived from the ancient Eastern discipline of yoga. You can find additional stretches that will be beneficial for your spine in books on yoga, and there are numerous excellent publications on this subject with photos and drawings demonstrating how to do the various stretches. A few are listed in the Appendix at the back of this book.

Yoga places great importance on the health of the spine, so if you are serious about overcoming your back problems, you will want to look into this fascinating subject further. Yoga classes are available in almost every major city throughout the Western world. Start with a class for beginners, and talk to the teacher beforehand about your specific back needs prior to enrolling.

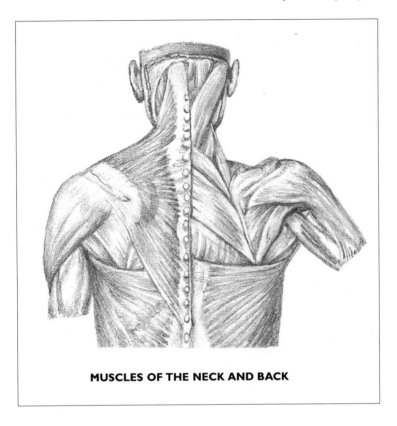

MUSCLES OF THE NECK AND BACK

Because we tend to bend slightly forward, such as when we are sitting, standing, or walking, over time, the back muscles will mold the bones of the spine into a bent-forward posture, getting worse as we get older. This puts more and more pressure and weight on the discs, rendering us more prone to serious back problems. We have all seen elderly people with bad backs bent over using canes to hobble along.

When the muscles in the back are healthy, strong, and flexible, they are able to maintain proper lumbar lordosis. Stretches involving gentle back bending can help restore a healthy posture for your back.

Finally, you can achieve a healthy posture and maintain a natural lordotic curve (see Chapter Two, page 21) in your spine by just being aware of your posture as often as you can. When this becomes an automatic habit, you will be able to maintain a correct and healthy posture, whether you are at rest, sitting, walking, or standing.

CHAPTER FIVE

Strengthening Your Back

THE SPINE IS OFTEN CALLED the backbone, a word that, not surprisingly, is also used to describe the foundation or most substantial part of anything. Your spine or backbone is your chief support in life, so it must be strong.

The term "spineless" is usually applied to a person who is lacking in courage or confidence. If you don't have confidence in your back, you will live in constant fear that it will go out. This fear will make you a prisoner of your back. It will cause you to develop an invalid mentality that will restrict your activities and put a damper on your entire life. Just as the mind affects the body, so the body affects the mind. By strengthening your back you can overcome fear and rebuild confidence in your back.

This chapter will provide you with exercises and activities for strengthening your back. But before starting a back-strengthening program, it is important to make sure that all injuries have had sufficient time to heal. For this, rest is required. After rest, comes stretching. With stretching comes greater oxygen delivery, increased blood flow, decongestion of stagnant fluids, and removal of waste products from the injured muscles, joints, discs, and vertebrae. After stretching, strengthening of the spine can be introduced.

Do not exercise immediately following a back injury or strain. Concentrate on stretching for the first two months, maybe longer. Walking can begin after you are up and about, but it must be done slowly at first. Be careful not to overdo it. Remember to allow your body time to heal and then build gradually. Slow and steady wins the race.

Strengthening involves the contracting of muscles, and when muscles contract, they exert a tremendous pulling force on the joints and opposing muscle groups. Over time, muscles that are repetitively contracted do get stronger, but they also get shorter and tighter and more stiff if they are not also systematically stretched. **Remember to stretch the muscles in your back before you do any strengthening activities or techniques, and while you are doing them.**

With strengthening activities comes the danger of subjecting your back to excessive forces, and doing further damage to it. For this reason, care must be taken to listen to your body at all times while doing strengthening exercises. By being careless and ignoring your body, it is easy to push too far and injure your back. I know; I have done it to myself many times in the past, and as a doctor, I'm supposed to know better!

Again, the stretching exercises described earlier also help to strengthen your back, so just by concentrating on the stretching alone, your back will become stronger. **Focusing on purely strengthening your spine should come only after full range of motion has been restored to your back through systematic stretching.**

Whatever methods or techniques you choose to adopt to strengthen your back, please remember to follow the principles outlined at the beginning of Chapter Four. In summary, they are:

+ Don't force or strain.

+ Don't ignore or push through the pain.

+ Pay attention to your breathing.

+ Listen to your body. If something doesn't feel right for your back, rest.

✦ Rest whenever you need to. Resting is not a sign of laziness or a characteristic of being a wimp. Resting is smart. Resting is healthy.

✦ Remember to rest periodically in the midst of your activities and busy days.

The exercises that strengthen your lower back involve the leg muscles, the gluteal muscles in the buttocks, the abdominal muscles, and, of course, the back muscles themselves. This is because the strongest and largest muscles, which are also the most critical for movement and mobility, are located in the lower half of your body.

Strengthening Your Leg Muscles

Strong leg muscles are very important to a healthy back. When legs are weak, too much stress is placed on the back causing back pain. This is especially true during lifting or strenuous activities.

When legs are strong, back problems diminish and usually disappear altogether. Most back pain patients I see, especially men, tend to carry more weight above the waist than below it, and the weight is not always fat. Quite often the person with back problems is muscular, athletic, and active, but has underdeveloped legs.

Walking, jogging, or cycling are simple exercises that develop general muscular strength in the legs. There are also other, more specific, exercises that target certain leg muscles.

STRENGTHENING YOUR CALVES AND THIGHS

The muscles in the calves and the quadriceps muscles in the thighs are critical to the support of the back. When calves and thighs are strong, they reduce the amount of work required by the back to support the weight of the body, as well as when lifting heavy loads. This is noticeable when standing, climbing stairs, getting out of bed in the morning, or getting up after sitting in a chair.

An excellent exercise for the calves is standing on your toes as described in the Mountain Pose (see page 112). A variation is to stand with your heels over the edge of a stair and come up on your toes as far as you can, then come back down lowering your heels as far as they will go. Try to build up slowly to 100 repetitions every day. After several weeks, you'll notice tremendous improvement in your back.

Strengthening Your Gluteal Muscles

The gluteal muscles in the buttocks also need to be firm and strong for a healthy back. They play a very important role in the support of the spine for standing, walking, running, and sitting. The Gluteal Squeezes described on page 78 can be incorporated into your daily routine as automatically as brushing your teeth. They will help your back immensely.

Strengthening Your Abdominal Muscles

The abdominal muscles are also vital to the health of the spine. Some experts actually consider them to be part of the spinal musculature. There is controversy, however, over how to strengthen them in a way that does not risk further damage or re-injury to the back, since abdominal exercises are often hard on the lower spine.

There are numerous exercises and regimens designed to strengthen the abdominal muscles. When you work on strengthening your abdominal muscles, try to make the movements slow and smooth, avoiding jerky, rapid motions that can strain your back. Here are a few suggestions:

+ **Sit-ups** can be modified to fit your particular needs; there are several variations. Remember to make all movements slowly and smoothly, and build from 5 repetitions a day for 1 or 2 weeks, to 10 repetitions. You can build systematically to as many as you want in this manner, but it would be better to limit yourself to 35 or a maximum of 50 sit-ups per day. Speed and quantity is not as important as quality and smoothness of execution. Remember to listen to your body.

✦ **Abdominal crunches** come in a variety of forms. They are like sit-ups done with bent knees and are easier on the spine than regular sit-ups. The same guidelines that apply to sit-ups apply to crunches when progressing in the number of repetitions you work up to.

✦ **Leg lifts** are also popular for strengthening the abdomen and back. They can be performed one leg at a time, which is safer for the back, or with both legs together. They can be done on the floor or on your bed or a sofa with your legs dangling off the side. Start with several repetitions of lifting one leg at a time for the first week, and then add slowly. Try doing both legs together after several weeks of lifting one leg at a time.

Remember to start all abdominal exercises with very few repetitions the first day. Wait a day to make sure there are no untoward effects on your back before proceeding. Add a few more repetitions each day until you have built your abdominal muscles up. Don't overdo it. If you get your abdominal muscles too tight from overstrengthening without stretching, they may pull your spine out of balance and strain your back.

Strengthening Your Back Muscles

Many important muscles in the back need to be strengthened. It is difficult to isolate each one, however, so the best approach is to strengthen them as a group, approaching the back from as many angles as possible.

The yogic system, originally from India, focuses on building up the strength and health of the spine from almost every conceivable angle, and is the most comprehensive back strengthening program I have discovered. I usually direct people who are serious about improving the health of their back to one or more of the numerous publications on this subject (see Appendix) or to a yoga class in their community.

Other conventional exercises for strengthening the back can also be helpful, but be sure to follow the precautions and guidelines outlined earlier in this chapter.

Awareness of Muscle Balance While Exercising

If one side of your body is weaker than the other, and it usually is, try to identify which is the weaker side of your body, then set out to deliberately strengthen it. Gradually increase the strength of the weaker side by favoring the muscles on your weak side as you exercise. This will allow your weak side to catch up to your stronger side and will help balance the muscular support in your back.

SIMPLE EXERCISES FOR STRENGTHENING YOUR BACK

You can strengthen your back by doing simple and practical exercises even in the midst of your daily activities. These can be done at home, at work, while you are having fun, relaxing, playing your favorite sport, or while going for a fitness workout at your local health club or gym.

I recommend the following activities and exercises to help strengthen your back and alleviate your back problems. This list, however, is not intended to be complete or all inclusive. You may have your own favorite exercise or strengthening regime that works well for you.

Walking
Walking should be one of the first, if not the first, exercise attempted after recovering from a back injury or back strain. It is the most nat-

ural exercise you can do. Most people can walk by one year of age, and continue to walk up until the time of death, which can sometimes extend beyond 100 years. Walking builds up the legs, as we've discussed, which are essential to support the spine. The stronger your legs, the more support there is for your back.

Keep the following points in mind as you begin walking:

+ Increase your distance and time slowly. Don't overdo it in the beginning. Start with just 5 minutes a day and then add 5 minutes each week until you can build to at least 30 minutes, 3-6 days a week. Find a speed that is comfortable for you. It is better to walk farther at a slower pace than to walk a shorter distance faster.

+ Try to maintain good posture as you walk. You may use a cane if it helps you.

+ After you've built to 30 minutes a day, try walking up hills as this will help develop the quadriceps muscles in your thighs. On level ground, try walking on your toes to strengthen your calves. Try to build to at least 30 minutes a day, 3-6 days a week.

Swimming

If you have access to a pool, ocean, lake, river, pond, or other body of water, and you like to swim, swimming can be an excellent exercise for building up the overall health of your back.

Because there is no weight on the spine when you are swimming, this reduces the risk of trauma, strain, or injury while you are strengthening the muscles that help support your back. Also, swimming involves a lot of stretching as you move your arms, legs, and back, so it can give you a good workout without tightening up the muscles in the back.

To build up the muscles in your lower spine, hips, buttocks, and legs, you will have to focus more on the kicking movements, which are usually everybody's weak spot. To build both awareness and strength in these muscles, you might want to try using swim fins. Here are a couple of other ideas that may be helpful:

✦ Start out by just treading water with your legs. This requires a scissor kick, which stretches and strengthens your hips, thighs, and lower back. Do this for several minutes or as long as you are able without tiring.

✦ Hold onto a wall, keep your legs straight, and then kick up and down making a splash each time you kick. Try to keep your knees straight and your awareness focused on your lower back. Find a speed that feels good for you, and kick for 10-15 minutes at a stretch before resting.

✦ Grab a kickboard and position your body and arms so that when you kick, your back is comfortable. Do either the up and down kick (freestyle or crawl kick) or the scissors (frog kick) with your awareness focused on your legs, hips, and lower spine as you do your laps.

If you make your arms do all the work and hardly kick at all, your upper body will develop and strengthen at the expense of your legs and lower body, and this will not help your back become stronger, although the swimming may be therapeutic for your heart, mind, and spirit. Because your leg muscles are more important than your arms in helping to support your spine and the weight of your body, it is important to focus on building them up.

You can try different strokes such as the breast stroke, back stroke, side stroke, or freestyle stroke. **Remember not to overdue or force or strain, and continue to stretch so you don't tighten-up.**

Jogging

A regular jogging program can be very helpful for your back and psychologically and spiritually rewarding, **if you regularly stretch your muscles**. This applies especially to the hamstrings (see page 32), which tend to tighten-up with running. Listen to your body and don't overdo it. Many joggers don't stretch enough. Their back and leg muscles end up being very, very tight, which sets them up for back problems.

Generally, jogging on softer surfaces, such as grass, dirt, and sand, is easier on the back and joints due to less jarring. Because these are often uneven surfaces, however, they may result in more foot and ankle injuries, so please take care.

If you decide to jog, try to start with as slow and comfortable a pace as possible, focusing on strengthening the weaker side of your body by deliberately favoring these muscles when you move your legs.

Keep the following guidelines in mind as you start a regular jogging program:

1. Start out jogging only after you can walk without back discomfort for at least 30 minutes a day.

2. Start out at a very slow pace. Jog only for 10 minutes the first day, then skip a day before jogging again for 10 minutes. Jog a maximum of 4 days a week for 2 weeks doing 10 minutes a day.

3. Always stretch before and after you jog. Concentrate on your hamstrings since jogging tightens these muscles.

4. Stretch on your days off. Again, concentrate on your hamstring muscles.

5. After 2 weeks, if all is well and there are no signs of discomfort in your back, begin jogging for 20 minutes, every other day. Stretch your hamstrings on your days off.

6. After 2 more weeks, you can build up to 30 minutes a day, 3-6 days a week. If you jog more than 30 minutes a day, the side effects may outweigh the benefits. If you are diligent on your stretching program, however, you may be able to jog longer and farther, and more often. This is entirely up to you.

Caution: If for some reason, jogging makes your back worse, either while jogging or the next day, then you've got to make some adjustments. Either cut back on the intensity, speed, or distance, or the number of times you jog each week. If none of these adjustments help, you may need to stop for awhile and concentrate more on stretching and other exercises that are compatible with your back's present condition. The key is to listen to your body and honor it. I had to wait five years after my surgery before I could resume a regular jogging program.

Cycling

Riding a bicycle, either stationary or moving, helps to build up the muscles in your legs, which help to support your spine. The only problem with cycling is that it usually entails sitting in a bent-over position. Sitting by itself can increase the pressure on the discs, and bending forward is even harder on the back.

If you enjoy bicycling, however, either on a stationary or regular bike, then try to adjust your seat and handlebars to minimize the bent-over position of your spine. When you begin bicycling after a back injury or strain, start with 5-10 minutes each day for 2 weeks, and then double the time if all is going well with your back. In the beginning, it is better to skip a day to rest and stretch in between cycling days. Every 2 weeks you can add 5-10 more minutes until you've built up to 30-40 minutes. Remember to stretch your hamstrings every day that you cycle and concentrate on the gentle back-bending stretches described in Chapter Four to counter the forward bending and sitting of cycling.

Weight-lifting

Many people injure their backs while weight-lifting, so it is with great caution that I recommend weight-lifting for building up and strengthening the muscles in your back.

Note: Back exercises done on weight machines or with free weights must be undertaken with great caution. Since these exercises focus mainly on the upper back, they are not as helpful for strengthening the more problematic lower spine, and may tighten the spine and work against developing more flexibility, which is one of your primary goals.

It can be helpful to regularly work on specific areas of your body, particularly your legs, using weights that don't add any stress or strain to your back. Weight exercises that focus on the thigh and calf muscles, when properly and safely executed, can be extremely helpful to build up the muscles in your legs that ultimately benefit the back. Use light weights and more repetitions. A physical therapist or personal trainer can assist you in finding the proper weights as you get started and can help you establish a regular routine that is safe and effective for your back.

When doing weight-lifting exercises, always be sure to:

+ Stretch on a daily basis to prevent the muscles from tightening up.

+ Start out with light weights and build up the strength of the muscles slowly. Again, a personal trainer or physical therapist can help you find the right weights in the beginning.

Machines tend to be safer than free weights because they move in a predictable track, are generally smoother, and have built-in safety features should you slip or lose your balance.

Whatever routine you choose, start light and build slowly and steadily. Remember not to force or strain. Take your time. Be patient in building up the strength of the muscles in your body and back. Remember to keep stretching.

Calisthenics and Aerobics
Some of these exercises can be fun and helpful to strengthening your legs and back. Music in the background adds an element of fun and relaxation.

Avoid jerky, jarring, rapid, sudden motions that may tweak your back muscles and cause them strain or injury. Try to move your body with grace and smoothness. If something doesn't feel right, don't do it. Listen to your body and remember to breathe!

Remember your stretching regimen. Don't work out in freezing cold, air-conditioned health clubs where your muscles haven't had time to warm up. A hot shower, jacuzzi, or massage can be a nice way to wind down from these exercises. Your back will appreciate these treats.

Your Favorite Sports

Sports are an excellent way to exercise and stay in shape. Studies have shown that people who devote themselves to at least one sport or hobby live longer and enjoy a much higher quality of life than those who don't. But sporting activities can sometimes be harmful to your back if you choose to ignore your body's messages in favor of questing for victory and glory. Personal triumph at the expense of your back is not worth it.

Tennis, golf, and skiing come to mind as lifelong sports that fit into this category, but it could also be sailing, polo, hiking, canoeing, or one of many others. Mine is surfing.

When participating in sports, remember to be conscious of your back at all times. Be kind to your back. Don't put it in a position of jeopardy. Don't risk injury for the sake of winning the game. In between the action, focus your awareness on your back and stay relaxed by breathing deeply and slowly. Don't force or strain in your effort to win.

The physical and psychological benefits of participating in your favorite sport have a positive effect on your spirits and overall health, well-being and, ultimately, your back.

If you have a debilitating back problem that is keeping you from doing what you truly enjoy, read *The Way of the Peaceful Warrior*. It is the true story of a college gymnast, Dan Millman, who crushed his leg so badly in a motorcycle accident that he was told by his doctors that he would never be able to compete again, or even walk without a limp. After initially becoming angry, depressed, and then hopelessly self-destructive, he somehow found inner strength and went on to win the Olympic Gold Medal in the trampoline. If your back is keeping you from doing something that you love to do, I recommend this book highly. It shows how a goal can motivate you to make the effort to heal your back.

You may not be able to do what it is you love now because of your back, but if you hold that goal in front of you, you are much more likely to be motivated to do the work that will take you back to it soon.

When you do come back to your favorite sport after a long lay-off due to an injury, you will appreciate participating more than ever before. A spirit of gratitude will permeate your being and you will play with more grace and style. You will be more precise and calculating in your movements. You will be smarter, wiser, and you will discover a deeper, inner aspect to the game that is more uplifting and personally enriching than the competitive thrill of winning.

It was like this for me and surfing. When my doctor told me I might not ever surf again after my operation, I was devastated. I imagined I'd never get back out into the ocean again, and I have loved the ocean since my mother first taught me how to bodysurf at the age of four.

I remember my first time back in the water. It felt so good to paddle back out through the waves on my surfboard. I can't describe the sense of exhilaration I felt. It was as if I'd been reborn, and life had given me a second chance. That day I surfed better than I can ever recall, and I didn't fall once. I continue to improve and enjoy surfing to this day.

Your favorite sport can be a big part of your life, even if you have had chronic back problems. You owe it to yourself to find a way to continue doing it so that it doesn't hurt your back and can actually help it. You may have to develop a different perspective or a new attitude or approach, but whatever it takes, get out there and do it. You'll be glad you did. If you need inspiration, tune in to the Special Olympics and don't forget *The Way of The Peaceful Warrior.*

Other Benefits to the Back from Exercising

In addition to strengthening your muscles, regular exercise benefits your back in other important ways.

Regular exercise has been shown to lead to weight loss. Weight loss decreases the stresses and strains on the spine, improves appearance and self-esteem, lifts spirits, and provides added energy to the body. With weight loss usually comes loss of abdominal belly fat which helps to improve posture and eases the pressure on the lower spine. It can also alleviate depression.

Exercise also improves cardiovascular health, with improved blood vessel tone and greater strength and endurance of the pumping muscles of the heart. This leads to increased blood flow to the back with greater oxygen and nutrient delivery to the tissues and cells of the spinal musculature. Increased blood flow also leads to improved removal of cellular metabolic waste products which also promotes the healing of your back.

A Final Word

If I could sum up the essence of this chapter in one phrase it would be this: Move it or lose it.

Movement is life, and when we stop moving certain parts of our body, muscles stiffen and weaken, joints freeze up, and pain increases when we apply a force of any kind to these areas. How we move, however, and when, is what I've attempted to describe in this chapter.

I would also add: Rest is best. It is important not to move too soon after a back injury or strain. In the acute phase of an injury, rest allows the tissues in your back to heal and repair themselves, which the body knows how to do if you give it the time and nourishment it needs. When you are over the acute phase of an injury or strain and are on to rehabilitating yourself through stretching and strengthening, knowing when to rest is very important.

There is an inherent rhythm in the workings of the universe and in nature that can help you appreciate the concept of timing when it comes to your back. Many people make the mistake of being too active too soon after a back injury and suffer relapse after relapse as a consequence. This is what happened to me over a 15-year period before I finally learned the hard way. It is important to understand the wisdom of patience.

Other people become so intimidated by their back pain that they refuse to move at all. These people haven't learned that the longer the inactivity, the harder it is to get back into the game.

It all boils down to knowing how much and when to move, when to rest, and for how long. If you make listening to your body a regular habit, and apply the techniques and information offered in this book so far, before you know it, you will be able to heal your back pain and enjoy a stronger, more flexible spine than ever before.

== CHAPTER SIX ==

Stress Management for Your Back

MOST BACK INJURIES and problems occur just preceding, during, or shortly after major periods of stress. If you want your back to heal, it is critical to learn how to relax and manage your stress. This is the most important part of the Back To Life Program.

In this chapter you will learn specific simple, yet powerful and effective stress management and relaxation techniques. They require no special technology, props, gadgets, or expensive electronic devices. All you need is your mind and body. They are easily learned and can be done in the convenience of your home or at work in the midst of your busy schedule.

Stress and Your Back

Science is just now beginning to verify what the ancients have long since known to be true: The mind and body are indeed connected. Understanding this mind-body connection will help you understand how stress works, how it affects your back, and how to help your back heal through stress management and relaxation techniques.

No one disputes that how you feel physically can affect your mental

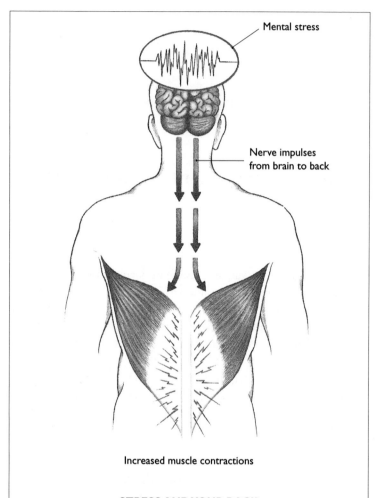

Mental stress

Nerve impulses
from brain to back

Increased muscle contractions

STRESS AND YOUR BACK

Stress activates and stimulates the nervous system...causing increased
muscle contractions, increased muscle tone and tension...which can
cause muscle spasms...leading to muscle strain, injury, and pain.

outlook. For example, everyone knows that even a common cold can dampen your spirits and darken your mood. But for most people it is not so obvious that the mind also influences the body.

Can what goes on inside your head really have an effect on your body? Experts say "yes." In fact, they have discovered that your mind exerts a much more powerful influence on your body than your body does on your mind. A good example of this is the influence of stress.

Stress gets passed down from your brain to your body through the far-reaching tentacles of the nervous system, whose presence can be felt by every organ and tissue in the body. The more stress, the more your nervous system is stimulated, and the more your body is affected. In particular, stress strongly affects the activities of the autonomic nervous system, that part of your nervous system that regulates all involuntary functions in your body, including your breathing, heart rate, blood pressure, body temperature, bladder and bowel function, resting muscle tone or tension, and many other important functions.

The autonomic nervous system consists of two branches, the sympathetic and parasympathetic systems. The sympathetic nervous system, highly sensitive to stress, tends to speed up metabolism and excite the body, while the parasympathetic slows down metabolism and induces relaxation in the body.

When stress enters your system, it activates the sympathetic nervous system, causing your muscles to automatically tense and tighten-up, which can have direct and painful consequences on your back. Long-term, unmanaged stress, experienced daily and repeated over weeks, months, or even years, can virtually cripple your back by causing devastating chronic muscle tension that distorts the normal alignment of the spine.

Stress management and relaxation help to reduce the activity of the sympathetic nervous system while strengthening the influence of the parasympathetic system. This causes all the muscles in your body to relax, including the muscles in your back, allowing your spine to return to its normal alignment.

Learning to Relax

For most of us, relaxation does not come easily because we were never taught how to do it. Unfortunately, we are paying dearly for our ignorance, as more and more of the diseases we suffer from, including heart disease, are linked to stress and anxiety.

Compelling evidence of our inability to relax lies in the inordinate amount of tranquilizers prescribed on a daily basis to people suffering from anxiety, stress, or tension-related disorders. A recent patient of mine, named Del, is a good example of this phenomenon.

Del was a 38-year-old laborer whose back had gone out two days prior to visiting me. He was worried that he wouldn't be able to work and put food on the table for his family. The more he thought about his predicament, the worse his back got. "The muscle spasms are unbelievable," he told me. "It feels like it's getting worse!"

In the course of taking a medical history, I asked Del if he knew how to relax, and if he did, how did he do it?

"Of course I know how to relax, Doc. When I finish at the job site, I come home to my wife and kids, shower-up, and sit down to two or three brews in front of the tube before dinner. I get so relaxed I often fall asleep in my reclining chair. This works for me every time," he replied.

I explained to Del that there was a better, more powerful way to relax that increased awareness and would not give him that hazy, sloppy mental feeling, or cause any damage to his liver the way alcohol does. Del agreed to try it out and it worked.

By learning how to truly relax, Del not only solved his back problem, he also feels more mentally alert and balanced throughout the day. And because he no longer zones-out when he comes home, his wife and kids enjoy being around him more.

While alcohol, drugs, food, and other substances may help you to relax *temporarily*, they have unhealthy side effects. They create dependence and can lead to addiction, since the body eventually develops tolerance to these things, and greater and greater quantities are required to create the desired effect. Eventually they don't work anymore, and actually end up creating more stress in your life.

There are much more powerful and natural ways to relax than taking tranquilizers, alcohol, or drugs, that are healthy, restorative, and healing. One of the most powerful, yet simple relaxation techniques comes from the yogic tradition of India and has been around for over a thousand years. Just minutes a day of this relaxation technique can be the equivalent of three hours sleep. It is so effective, we call it deep relaxation.

How Deep Relaxation Heals Your Back

Deep relaxation is a powerful mind-body technique that can ease your pain almost instantaneously by relaxing those tight, congested, knotted, spasming, painful muscles. It helps these muscles loosen their grip, creating a space so your back can breathe, stretch, and move a little. The healing process begins almost immediately as increased blood flow brings more nourishment and oxygen to the cells of the choked and suffocating muscles.

Deep relaxation works through the autonomic nervous system, ridding the body of stress, anxiety, and tension. It works on the mental level by reducing agitation and quieting the mind, which in turn, reduces activity in the sympathetic nervous system while activating the parasympathetic system. You'll recall that reduced sympathetic nervous system activity, along with increased parasympathetic activity, helps to relax your muscles, allowing them to release chronic tension that has often been stored up for years.

Here's how deep relaxation works:

When muscles relax, they lengthen. This allows the tiny blood vessels in the muscles that were previously compressed to open up. Improved blood flow to the muscles results in a decongestion of the tissues in the area. Inflammation and swelling, hallmarks of both acute and chronically injured backs, reduces, resulting in healing.

Improved blood flow provides greater oxygen delivery, better nutrition, and more efficient removal of toxins to and from the muscles. Injured and diseased joints can now begin to heal. This is a direct, physiological result of relaxation, no matter how badly injured or painful your back may be.

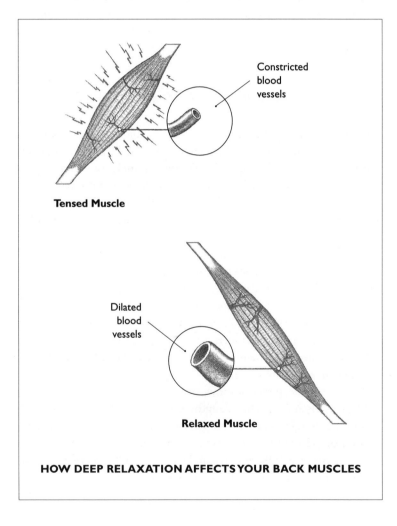

Constricted blood vessels

Tensed Muscle

Dilated blood vessels

Relaxed Muscle

HOW DEEP RELAXATION AFFECTS YOUR BACK MUSCLES

BENEFITS OF DEEP RELAXATION

Deep relaxation not only heals your back, it helps reduce the risk of recurrent back injuries. A stiff, tense spine is much more susceptible to injury than a flexible one, and learning to relax will help keep the muscles of your back soft and flexible. This will help you avoid injury and/or further damage to your back from physical trauma such as a fall, a blow, or from lifting a heavy object.

Because stress affects both the mind and the body, deep relaxation, which works on both levels, is especially effective for healing painful back conditions that have occurred during times of significant stress. When your body is relaxed, it exerts a calming and stabilizing influence on your mind. When your mind is relaxed, it exerts a powerful tranquilizing and relaxing effect on your body. When both mind and body are relaxed, stress is released and healing occurs. This is why deep relaxation is such a powerful mind-body technique for your back. Larry, a patient of mind with back problems, found out just how effective deep relaxation can be.

One day in Hawaii, where Larry lives, he was standing on a ladder cleaning the blades of the overhead fan in his living room. His parents would be arriving shortly from the mainland, and he was feeling anxious. He was expected to not only entertain them, but play tour guide as well, driving them all over the island.

With these thoughts in his head, it was no wonder that Larry momentarily lost his balance and fell. He felt his back go out even before he hit the floor.

When he came into my office the next day, he was in agony. "Can this be a chronic problem, or what, Doc?" he asked. "I don't feel like I'm accident prone, but this is my third injury in less than three months and I'm beginning to wonder. Just what do you think is going on here? It seems that my back goes out at the most inopportune times. I'm at my wit's end."

I explained to Larry the connection between his mind and body, and how stress, anxiety, and tension can affect the muscles of the spine, making them more susceptible to injury, spasm, and strain. "Stress is affecting your back, and that's why it's giving out when you need it the most," I explained.

Larry was incredulous. "Come on, Doc, gimme a break."

"It's true," I continued. "The constant bombardment of tense and anxious thoughts is inundating your nervous system with noxious impulses. These impulses reach your muscles and keep them in a constant state of contraction, rendering them tight and stiff. When your spine is tight and rigid, even a sneeze or bending down to tie a shoelace can throw it out of alignment for weeks and even months at a time. I have experienced these things over the 20-year course of my own back problems," I reminded him.

"They say the time to relax is when you can't afford to," I joked with Larry, but underneath my jovial tone I was dead serious.

I prescribed some muscle relaxants for the first few days of Larry's pain along with a prescription for deep relaxation to be done daily, which is a much more natural way to relax the muscles in the spine and has a more lasting effect. I gave him an audiocassette tape with my voice-guided, deep relaxation process that I'm about to describe to you.

When he returned to my office a week later, Larry was a new man. Although the pain wasn't completely gone, he had a calm and confident look on his face that told me he finally understood how to handle his back problems.

The more you regularly practice deep relaxation, the more benefits you will experience — benefits that extend far beyond your spine. Once you've experienced this deep state of relaxation, you will notice improvement in the following areas of your health:

✦ You will feel more relaxed throughout each day and will achieve inner poise. You will feel peaceful from within. You will know first-hand what it's like to be calm, cool, and collected like your favorite action-movie heroes, even under difficult circumstances.

✦ You will experience the feeling of being centered, and know that this is your true, natural state of being. You will learn to recognize when you are off-center and will be able to quickly correct it doing deep relaxation.

+ You will become much more aware of stressful situations and their effects on your body. While some stress in life may seem inevitable, you will learn how to avoid unnecessary stress.

+ You will become much more conscious of the harmful consequences of such emotions as fear and anger. You will learn how prolonged mental and emotional agitation can cause painful muscle tension and affect your spine adversely.

+ You will become much more aware of how the mind affects the body with its thoughts and activities, as well as vice versa.

+ You will have more energy throughout your day. You will be less stressed, more relaxed, and it will take much more to ruffle your feathers than before.

+ If you are prone to high blood pressure, you will see it normalize after some time. You may see other medical conditions improve as well.

+ If you suffer from anxiety, phobias, or even depression, you will see improvement in these areas.

   Deep relaxation is a simple technique, but don't let its simplicity fool you; it is a powerful tool for healing and taking away incapacitating back pain.

PRACTICING DEEP RELAXATION

For maximum benefit, especially when you are in significant pain, I recommend doing deep relaxation twice a day for 20-30 minutes at a time. If your pain is only minor, then once a day should suffice. The more you practice, the more proficient you'll become. The more you experience what it feels like to be relaxed, the more you will be able to maintain this calm state throughout the day, even in stressful situations. You will discover that what set you off before is not nearly as upsetting to you now. This will be a tremendous load off your back.

You can practice deep relaxation practically anytime throughout your day. About the only time that it isn't recommended is when you are driving or operating heavy equipment. You might relax so much that you fall asleep and cause an accident.

You don't have to lie down to practice deep relaxation, although it seems to be much more effective this way. Lying down completely takes the weight off your spine and gives it a much-needed rest. If your back hurts when you lie down, try placing pillows, blankets, or bolsters under your knees, or anywhere that will make it more comfortable for you. Find a comfortable position, making any modifications that are necessary so that the pain in your back won't be so intense that it distracts your mind from practicing this technique.

Follow these simple steps:

✦ Secure a 20-30 minute time slot for yourself where you can be completely alone, undisturbed, and quiet. Find a room where you can preferably close the door and be free from all distractions. Tell your family, loved ones, and significant others not to bother you and that you need to have this time by yourself. *It is important that no one disturb you until you are finished.* If you can't find a quiet place at all, use headphones or earplugs to help shut out any noise that might bother you. Take the phone off the hook or turn down the ringer so you can't hear it. Turn the lights down low.

✦ Now find a comfortable place to lie down on the floor or your bed. Place a blanket, quilt, or bedspread beneath you for padding if you need it. Use pillows under your head, knees, hips, or back in any way that is necessary for you to feel comfortable. Take your time and adjust yourself so that you feel you can be in this position for at least 20 minutes. If you can't get comfortable on your back, try rolling onto your side, placing pillows or blankets for support as needed. One side may be more comfortable than the other. Or you can lie on your stomach, placing a pillow under your hips, turning your head to the side, and resting your forehead on your folded arms. *Make sure there is no tension or strain on any of your joints, and that your arms, hands, legs, and feet are relaxed.*

Note: Before you proceed, you may want to get a small tape recorder and record your voice as you read the next section out loud. When the tape is finished recording, lie down, listen, and follow the words that you have just recorded. As an alternative, you might want to read the entire section before proceeding with the technique.

✦ Now gently close your eyes and bring your awareness into your body, focusing on the gentle movement of your breath as it flows down your chest and into your stomach and abdomen. You will notice a gentle up and down motion of your stomach and abdomen. Every time the breath flows into your body, your stomach and abdomen rise up and expand; every time the breath flows out of your body, your stomach and abdomen fall. Without trying to control the rate or depth of this motion, just allow your shoulders and body to relax as you observe this gentle, rhythmical movement. Allow your mind to relax and observe passively, without any effort or strain whatsoever.

✦ Imagine that every time you breathe in, you are breathing in life-sustaining oxygen to every cell and tissue in your body. Every time you breathe out, you are releasing carbon dioxide and tension, and are becoming more relaxed.

✦ Proceeding in this way, bring your awareness to the tips of your toes, to the bottom of your feet, the top of your feet, your heels, and your ankles. Take a nice, slow, deep breath, hold it for just a second after filling your lungs completely, then exhale slowly, smoothly, and fully as you allow all of these parts of your body to relax.

✦ Continue this way on up through your lower legs, your calf muscles, your knees, the backs of your knees, your thighs, the backs of your thighs, your hips, groin, buttocks, pelvic muscles, and lower spine.

✦ Focusing your awareness at the lower spine, notice how your back moves ever so slightly with each movement of your breath. Your breath can actually gently massage the muscles in your back this way. The greater the amount of breath you take in, the greater the movement of the muscles in your back.

   You will also notice that every time your abdomen and stomach rise up and expand, there is a gentle pulling motion on your spine. This helps to stretch and loosen any tight muscles in this area. You might notice a slight pain in your back as you do this. Don't worry; it will soon pass. Breathing out will allow those same muscles to release their grip and relax. In this manner, your back will loosen up and relax at the same time. This conscious breathing alone can result in tremendous reduction in pain when practiced for only 20-30 minutes at a time. The relief can be almost instantaneous.

✦ Next move your awareness to the middle of your back, your chest, upper back, and the area between your shoulder blades. Take a deep breath and then as you exhale completely, release all tension from these parts of your body and allow them to relax.

✦ Now allow your shoulders to feel very, very heavy, as if they weighed 2,000 lbs each. Allow them to just melt into the surface beneath you. Take a deep breath, exhale completely as you release all tension from your shoulders and let them relax.

✦ In a similar manner, relax your arms, elbows, forearms, wrists, hands, fingers, and fingertips.

✦ Next relax your neck, the back of your neck, the back of your head, the top of your head, and relax your forehead completely.

✦ Relax the muscles around your eyes, ears, and jaw. Relax all the muscles on your face, then bring a slight smile to your lips, stretching the more than 100 muscles it takes to make a smile.

✦ Release and relax all the muscles in your body, as you bring your awareness to the tip of your nose, where your breath is flowing in and out of your body through your nostrils.

✦ Without force or strain, observe this gentle flowing of the breath as if it were something different from yourself. Continuing on this way, allow yourself to let go and experience the wonderful feeling of complete relaxation. Be with this feeling for as long as you like.

✦ When you feel ready, slowly stretch your arms, legs, and spine, gently open your eyes, and give yourself time to adjust your awareness back to your surroundings as you prepare to resume your normal activities.

Congratulations! You have just experienced deep relaxation. That's really all there is to it, and it can change your life.

Continue practicing deep relaxation even after your back feels better. You wouldn't stop brushing your teeth if you didn't have any cavities. Your spine deserves the best possible care in the world, and deep relaxation, practiced on a regular basis, rescues you from immediate back pain, and it will also keep you out of trouble for good. Pete, one of my recent back pain patients, found this out.

Pete came into my office for a follow-up visit a week after a painful back injury. As I saw him move from the reception area and head for the examining room, I noticed that he was walking much straighter and with a brisker pace. Without even examining him, I could tell that he was better. "Doc, you were so right. The relaxation made all the difference in the world. When I first lay down to try it, I must admit

I was very skeptical. It seemed there was nothing to it, no substance, you know? It was just too simple, too easy. What could be so healing about watching my breath and lying down on my back? But you know, something kicked in when I was lying there and I was passively observing my breath. My mind just sort of settled down and for the first time in my life I felt I was truly aware of my body, as if I had discovered a long lost friend. It was a revelation! I'm so grateful. On top of that, within minutes the pain started to ease up for the first time in weeks. Now I feel I can see the light at the end of the tunnel! I have finally learned how to really relax!"

Note: If you fall asleep during deep relaxation, do not worry. It probably just means that your body is tired and overworked. Recent studies indicate that the vast majority of people suffer from varying degrees of sleep deprivation. Sleep deprivation is one of the factors that contributes to stress.

Breathing and Healing

Your breath is the link between your mind and your body. It is a well-known clinical fact that when a person is mentally agitated, anxious, or under stress of any kind, their breathing is disturbed. In these cases the breath is usually rapid and shallow. When the stress or anxiety becomes more severe, escalating into a full-blown panic attack, hyperventilation occurs. With hyperventilation, a person first begins to feel light-headed. Then numbness and tingling in both arms set in. Eventually, the person may even pass out from too little carbon dioxide in the blood. This is a condition seen commonly by doctors in emergency rooms around the world. The treatment is simply to slow down the breath, usually by placing a paper bag over the person's mouth. After several minutes, the symptoms go away and the person feels normal again.

Most of the time you go about the activities in your day without any awareness of your breath, but the simple fact is that without your breath, you couldn't live. Your body depends on the continuous flow of oxygen delivered from your lungs through the bloodstream into every cell and tissue.

Improvement in your health occurs when you become more aware of your breath and you practice simple breathing techniques. With improved breathing comes increased oxygenation of the blood. This means greater oxygen delivery to the muscles of your back, which promotes healing and strengthening. As your breath becomes more efficient, smooth, and relaxed, there is a calming effect on your brain and nervous system, reducing overall body tension. The muscles in your back become relaxed and your pain subsides.

BREATH AWARENESS FOR RELAXATION

Here is a simple, very effective technique for increasing awareness of your breath and inducing relaxation:

+ Lie down on your back, side, or stomach as you did for deep relaxation (see page 176). If you are able, you may sit with your back supported by a wall, the back of a chair, or any firm surface. Get in a comfortable position. Use pillows, blankets, or bolsters as needed so that your body is comfortable. It is important to get comfortable before you begin, otherwise your body will be a source of distraction for your mind.

   Note: The following sections can be read aloud into a tape recorder and then played back with your own voice acting as your guide, or you can read the sections in their entirety and then do the breathing, applying what you have read.

+ Now gently close your eyes and slowly breathe in. Direct your attention to the gentle up and down motion of your stomach and abdominal area. Notice how when the breath flows into your body, your stomach and abdomen rise up, and when the breath flows out of your body, your stomach and abdomen fall. Without trying to control the rate or depth of this movement, allow your mind to be a passive observer of this gentle up and down motion. Let your mind gently drift in and out of your body with your breath for about 3-5 minutes.

✦ Now, as you continue to keep your eyes closed, gently shift your awareness to the tip of your nose, where the breath is flowing in and out of your body through your nostrils. Once again, adopt a passive attitude, watching the breath move in and out of your body as if it were something different from yourself.

With your awareness focused at the tip of your nose, you may be able to detect a slight temperature difference between the warmer air that is leaving your body, and the cooler air that is entering your body. If you can, just notice the difference. Keep your awareness at this place, watching the breath flow in and out of your body, like the ebb and flow of the tides in the ocean or waves gently lapping up on a quiet, sandy seashore. Maintain this relaxed and passive focus for a few minutes.

✦ Next allow your awareness to follow the breath inside of your body. Feel the breath filling your lungs, expanding your chest and moving your stomach and abdomen up and down. From here, visualize and feel the breath entering into your bloodstream and nourishing every cell in your body with life-sustaining oxygen, from the tips of your toes to the top of your head and into your fingers and fingertips. Relax.

✦ Hold your awareness in these places as you continue to observe your breath. As you do this, allow all the muscles in your body to relax, and notice how good this feels. Continue to be with your breath this way for 5-10 minutes.

✦ When you are ready, bring your awareness back to the gentle up and down movement in your stomach and abdomen, watching as the breath continues to flow in and out of your body.

✦ Now, slowly open your eyes, stretch your body, and return to your normal activities.

THREE-PART BREATHING

This is another very simple, yet powerful, breathing technique for your back. It quiets your mind, relaxes your nervous system, and heals the muscles in your back by increasing the oxygen content in the blood, providing greater energy and vitality to your spine.

✦ Lie down on your back in a comfortable position. Bend your knees if this is more comfortable, placing pillows under your knees, hips, neck, or anywhere else that makes you comfortable.

✦ Gently close your eyes and slowly draw in a deep, full breath, feeling your stomach and abdomen expand fully as the breath enters into your body.

✦ Continue to draw in the breath until your stomach and abdomen are expanded to capacity, and without pausing, slowly exhale until your stomach and abdomen are completely empty. Even though you are taking larger than normal breaths, make sure the movement of the breath is smooth and fluid, and that you are not forcing or straining.

✦ On your next deep breath in, fully expand your abdomen and stomach to maximum capacity. Then feel the breath expand into your chest and rib cage fully. Feel your chest and rib cage lifting and expanding with the movement of the breath.

✦ Without pausing, slowly exhale by first emptying your chest and

rib cage and then emptying your stomach and abdomen completely. Make sure the movement of the breath is smooth and flowing, and that even though you are taking larger than normal
breaths, you are comfortable and are not forcing or straining in
any way. Try breathing this way for a minute or two until you are
familiar with this pattern.

+ On your next slow, deep inhalation, after filling your stomach and
abdomen to capacity and then your chest and rib cage, gently shift
your awareness to your shoulders and feel them slightly raising and
lifting as you draw the last of the breath slowly and deeply into this
part of your body.

+ When you are ready to exhale, relax and release your breath, allowing it to flow first out of your shoulder area, then your chest
and rib cage, then finally your stomach and abdomen. Empty your
breath completely from each of these parts of your body before
moving on to the next one. Even though you are taking deeper
than normal breaths, make sure the breath is flowing smoothly and
that you are relaxed, comfortable, and not straining.

+ After breathing like this for several minutes, return to normal
breathing and relax. Notice how your body feels. Notice how your
back feels. See if you can appreciate that your mind and nervous
system are calmer and you feel more centered.

BREATHING WITH SOUND

This is another powerful breathing technique derived from the yogic
tradition of India. It calms the mind, soothes the nerves, and helps to
relax the muscles in the body, particularly those that support the spine.

+ Sit or lie down in a comfortable position. Make sure that you find
a position you can remain in without discomfort for 10 or 15 minutes. Use pillows, blankets, bolsters, or any other form of support

you need. If your back is in pain, it might be easier to lie down and gently bend your knees, placing pillows or blankets under your legs so that you are comfortable.

+ Open your mouth and breathe in. Now breathe out, and gently say the sound *aahh*.

+ On your next breath, whisper the sound *aahh* and feel a gentle vibration coming from the region of your vocal cords in your throat.

+ Now close your mouth and breathe through your nose as you continue to make this whispering sound. You should be able to feel a slight grating sound coming from your vocal cords in the area of your throat.

+ Breathe in as slowly and as smoothly as you can, reducing the volume of the grating sound to less than a whisper, making it barely audible to anyone but you.

+ As you continue to breathe in and out slowly and smoothly, focus your awareness on this gentle grating sound as your breath flows in and out of your body. Continue to breathe with sound through both the inhalation and exhalation cycles of each breath for about 3-5 minutes.

+ After you have finished, remain with your eyes closed for a few more moments and relax, noticing a calm feeling within. Practicing breathing with sound for just 5 minutes a day will make a big difference in the health and healing of your back.

Visualization/Mental Imagery for the Spine

Visualization or mental imagery is a process that makes use of the fact that our minds and brains like to think in terms of images. This can be summed up in the saying, *A picture is worth a thousand words.* If you can form a picture in your mind, it is easy to understand and grasp a concept. Get the picture?

Visualization or mental imagery is something everyone experiences on a daily basis, without even being aware of it. For example, when your children borrow the family car and don't return it on time, you worry that they have gotten into an accident, and form a mental picture of the accident scene. You can almost see, hear, and smell the images. There is a lot of broken glass. There is blood on the windshield. The ambulance lights are flashing. Someone is being taken away in a stretcher. In the blink of an eye, you have seen, reviewed, and processed the entire scene in your mind.

Daydreaming is another example of how you form mental images of an incident that might happen or might have happened, or of a place where you wish you were or where you have actually been. While you are in the state of daydreaming, the images of the experience feel quite real to you. Sexual fantasies are another example of how you use your mind to project images of events or people into your consciousness.

Physiological changes in your body can accompany these images; that's how real they seem. This is because the brain always converts these images, real or imagined, into electrical impulses before transmitting them to the body via the nervous system. The body can't distinguish between real or imagined images and responds the same way to both.

Harmful as well as beneficial physiological changes can occur in your body through the mental pictures formed by the brain. Worrying is known to cause ulcers, which can cause internal bleeding and even death if they are allowed to go untreated. This is because the stressful pictures that circulate in your mind when you worry cause electrical impulses to be sent to your stomach that cause the cells in the stomach to secrete digestive acid. If enough acid is produced over time, it can burn a hole in your stomach or small intestines, resulting in a bleeding ulcer. Worrisome images produced by your mind can cause spasm in your coronary arteries and lead to a heart attack. In the same way, you can develop high blood pressure and a host of other ailments including back pain.

You can use the natural imaging language of your mind to help heal your back. I would like to introduce you to several visualization/imagery techniques that are very easy to do and have helped many people who once had bad backs. These are the very same techniques I learned to use to overcome my own back problems.

IMAGING A STRONG AND FLEXIBLE SPINE

✦ Get in a comfortable position and relax your mind and body as you did for deep relaxation and breath awareness. Close your eyes and use your breath to help you relax.

✦ Now allow an image to form in your mind of your back as you would like it to be—strong, vibrant, healthy, energetic, flexible, and alive. See your back bending in all directions with suppleness and vigor. See it move with grace and precision. See yourself involved in your favorite activities making unrestricted movements with your back feeling strong and flexible. See the muscles in your back rippling with strength as they support you during the most vigorous and fun activities you can imagine. Hold these images in your mind as you breathe deeply into them.

✦ Breathe these images into your whole body and then into your back. Allow their energy to merge with your back. Stay with these images as you breathe life into them. Allow your back to absorb the qualities and characteristics of your images.

✦ Release these images from your mind whenever you desire, but know that you can call them up again whenever you choose.

✦ The more often you picture how you would like your back to be, the more vivid and lifelike you can make your images, the more your back will take on their characteristics, and the faster it will heal.

187

This technique will send electrical impulses from the brain, through the nervous system, and to your back where it will actually transform your body's physiology. Remember, the body cannot tell the difference between real or imagined images, since it receives its messages from the brain through the nervous system in the form of electrical impulses. If you can temper your desire to heal with a little patience and perseverance, soon your images will translate into reality.

ANIMAL IMAGING

+ Imagine an animal with a strong back, such as a horse, cow, elephant, or rhinoceros, or one with a flexible spine, such as a python, cobra, crocodile, or salamander. Form a picture of this animal in your mind.

+ Now close your eyes, relax, and breathe deeply. As you feel yourself relaxing, allow the image of the animal to come into clearer focus.

+ Visualize the qualities of this animal's back that you would like to incorporate into your own spine. Hold onto this image for as long as possible, breathing slowly and gently, and remaining relaxed. See your back becoming like the back of this animal.

+ Release this mental picture and open your eyes after you have done this visualization.

Repeat this visualization as often as you are able. It only takes 10-15 minutes at a time. Know that your back can and will take on these characteristics if you hold onto an inspiring image over time. You can also keep pictures around your house, car, or workplace to remind you of this animal.

When I was working on my back, I chose to image a horse. Because I lived near horses, I would actually place my hand on the back of a horse and imagine that my back was becoming stronger and healthier. On days that I was in severe pain, this technique would completely take it away.

This is a very helpful technique when your back muscles are experiencing intense spasms and you can feel them forming into tense and painful knots. You will feel considerable pain relief from doing this exercise in just 10-15 minutes.

+ Get in a comfortable position, close your eyes, breathe slowly and deeply, and relax.

+ Allow an image to form of your back and how you perceive it to be at this very moment.

+ Now imagine a pair of soft and comforting hands massaging your stiff and sore back muscles from inside your body. Imagine every single muscle fiber in your back being gently caressed, rubbed, massaged, and loved by the most wonderful pair of healing hands in the world.

+ As you breathe in, feel these hands gently squeezing and rubbing on the most painful, knotted-up areas of your muscles.

+ As you breathe out, feel the hands and muscles relax as the soreness and tension from your tight and stiff muscles dissipates with the expulsion of your breath.

+ Once again, as you breathe in, feel the hands gently squeezing and rubbing out the kinks and knots of your painful and spasming back muscles. As you breathe out, feel the tension and pain releasing.

Continue to synchronize the breathing with your imagery for several minutes, relaxing your entire body and your spine as you do this exercise.

Dialoguing With Your Back Pain

Dialoguing is a technique that can provide you with valuable information from your body's own healing system. Important insights can result from the process of dialoguing with your symptoms, using the language of imagery to mediate between your subconscious mind and your back.

I found this technique very helpful for getting to know why my back was hurting, what I was doing wrong, how to correct it, and what it needed to heal. From dialoguing, I also discovered that my physical pain had much deeper emotional roots, which I explored and resolved successfully with this process.

To learn how to dialogue with your pain, follow these simple steps:

✦ Be in a comfortable position. Close your eyes and relax, taking a slow, deep breath in as you focus your awareness on your back. Try to feel your back from within, noticing the gentle movement of your breath as it flows in and out of your body.

✦ When you feel ready, think of your back pain and allow an image to form in your mind that would represent it if it were to take on the shape and form of an image. Don't have any expectations of what this image should look like. Just allow the first image that comes into your mind to be as it is, even if at first it is not very clear. This may seem strange, and nothing might come into your mind for a few minutes, but if you can just stay with your pain, keep your mind focused within, and continue to relax your body and be aware of your breathing, you will be surprised to see that an image eventually does form. It may not be a visual image; it may be a sound or a tactile sensation, but you can expect an image of some sort to form and come into focus. Once an image does form, keep your body relaxed and breathe deeply as you allow that image to come into clearer focus.

✦ Continue to breathe and remain relaxed as you focus on your image. Notice the shape of the image, what color it is, what texture it is, and any other qualities you may observe. If the image is far away and seems nebulous or indistinct in your mind's eye, either move yourself closer to the image or move the image closer to you until you feel comfortable. The image may change and evolve into a variety of shapes or colors at any time throughout the process or it may remain fixed. Whatever happens, try to keep your mind open and nonjudgmental.

✦ When the image has stabilized, try to initiate a dialogue with it. Introduce yourself to the image as if it has its own personality and the ability to communicate with you. In reality, it actually does, since it is connected to your own innate intelligence. You can ask the image if it has a name and see if it replies. This will help facilitate a dialogue.

✦ Whatever name first comes to you, accept it and use it. Address your image with respect, just like you would a person you'd never met before. Carry on a normal conversation, only do so silently in your mind. This may seem silly initially, but if you stick with the process, you will find this technique to be extremely valuable in gaining specific information and insights on how to heal your back.

✦ Direct your questions to your image and wait for the appropriate responses. For instance, you might want to ask the image of your back pain what purpose it is serving. Why is it there? Why does it hurt so much? How long will it take to go away? What can you do to diminish its intensity? You can ask the image anything you want that you feel might help heal your back and make your pain go away.

✦ At any time during this process, you can move closer to your image if you feel like it. You can also step into and merge with your image when and if the time feels right.

✦ When you feel you have gotten all the information you need from this process, or when you feel you'd like to close the dialogue, express your gratitude to your image, say goodbye, and know that you can meet again at any time you choose. Take a deep breath and slowly open your eyes when you feel ready.

✦ You may want to write down any insights or specific information you gained from this experience. Know that you can repeat this internal dialogue whenever you like. The more you do it, the easier it becomes, and the more insights and information you will acquire to help you heal your back.

There are many good books and tapes on these and other visualization and imagery techniques. Some are listed in the Appendix.

Meditation for Stress Management

Meditation is a powerful technique that promotes healing. It calms and centers the mind, promotes mental tranquility, soothes and relaxes the nervous system, and reduces muscle tension in the back.

Meditation is a state of relaxation and heightened mental awareness that occurs when your mind is quiet, calm, and focused. It is not mystical or magical. It is very natural and ordinary, and it feels good. We have all experienced meditation at one time or another in our lives, even if only for a few brief moments.

Meditation happens when your mind is fully absorbed in the present moment. This occurs when you are not thinking about the past or the future, and you are just aware of what is happening in the here and now.

When children play, they are so intent on their playing that they are not aware of anything else. They are not aware of the past or the future; they are only aware of their playing. They get angry when you call them in to eat dinner because you are disturbing their play. They may be hungry, but they forget about food because they are so absorbed in what they are doing. The same is true of meditation; it is total absorption in the present moment.

There are many techniques for meditation. You will probably want to try several before selecting at least one that you can embrace as your own. Two very simple meditation techniques are described here.

DRIFTING THOUGHT-CLOUDS MEDITATION

This is a simple meditation technique that you can do in just several minutes. It even works when you are in extreme pain. You can do this while lying down with your legs straight or bent, pillows under your knees, or in a seated position on the floor or in a chair, whichever is more comfortable for your back. Make sure your entire body is comfortable and that you will be able to stay in this position for at least 5-10 minutes.

+ Close your eyes and breathe slowly and deeply. After several breaths, gradually shift your awareness to your stomach and abdomen, noticing the gentle up and down movement that occurs with the movement of your breath.

+ As you remain focused on the movement of your stomach and abdomen, continue to observe your breath as it flows in and out of your body, relaxing your shoulders and back as you do this.

+ Now shift your awareness to the tip of your nose where your breath is flowing in and out of your body. Keeping your body relaxed, allow your breath to move at its own rate and rhythm. Let your mind relax, observing the movement of your breath as if it were something different from yourself.

✦ As you continue to focus your awareness on the movement of your breath, you may notice certain thoughts that come into your mind. Don't try to hold on to these thoughts, but rather just observe them as they come and go. Imagine they are like clouds drifting by.

✦ Now imagine that you are lying down or sitting in a room with high walls and windows, and these clouds, which represent your thoughts, are gently drifting in and out through the open windows in the room.

✦ Continue to see your thoughts as clouds, observing them passively as they flow in and out of the room. As you do this, continue to breathe in slowly and gently.

✦ Allow your thought-clouds to drift by without any need to respond or attend to them.

✦ Feel your mind releasing tension as you release your thoughts, becoming more relaxed and focused with each breath.

✦ Feel your back becoming more relaxed.

✦ After 5-10 minutes, slowly open your eyes and return your awareness to your immediate surroundings when you are ready.

Do this meditation whenever you feel yourself becoming anxious or tense, when you are in pain, or every day to prevent these uncomfortable sensations. This is a very pleasant and uplifting meditation that leaves you feeling inspired and refreshed.

HEALING IMAGES OF NATURE MEDITATION

We all know how healing nature can be. Today's popular health writers are extolling nature's virtues as a powerful healing force while more and more doctors regularly prescribe frequent, close, therapeutic encounters with nature for their ailing patients.

When you can't be outside in your favorite place in nature and you want to relax or uplift your spirits, this meditation will help you get there. You will find it very tranquilizing for your mind and healing to your back. This type of meditation incorporates the use of imagery.

+ Lie down or sit in a comfortable position. Make sure you are comfortable enough to be able to maintain this position for 10–15 minutes. Use pillows, bolsters, or blankets for support if needed. Try to keep your spine straight.

+ Close your eyes and direct your awareness within, feeling the gentle movement of your breath as it flows in and out of your body.

+ Relax your shoulders, your spine, and all the muscles in your body as you continue to observe the movement of your breath.

+ Allow an image to form in your mind of a beautiful forest and woods. See yourself walking in these woods along a quiet path. Continue to breathe as your image comes into clearer focus.

+ As you walk along the path in the woods, see yourself suddenly come upon a small clearing that opens into a lush, green meadow with beautiful, delicate, multi-colored wildflowers in full bloom.

+ Notice the sunlight streaking through the tree branches and surrounding foliage, illuminating the wildflowers and meadow, bathing them in a soft light.

+ Hear the birds echoing their melodic songs across the meadow from high up in the treetops.

+ Breathe in deeply, noticing how fresh and alive it seems, filled with the scents of the wildflowers and surrounding woods. Linger for a few moments here, slowly breathing in this lovely fragrance.

✦ Notice that near a corner of the meadow there is a small stream passing through. It is making a gentle gurgling sound. Pause for a moment and listen quietly. Relax; you are not in a hurry!

✦ Breathe in deeply and allow yourself to be fully immersed in this beautiful scene, drinking in all the sights, sounds, and smells around you. Relax.

✦ After 5–10 minutes, when you are ready, take a deep breath, let the images fade, and slowly open your eyes. After you have opened your eyes, try not to jump into your next activity right away, but rather remain in the present moment for awhile, without thinking about the past or worrying about the future. Give yourself permission to feel calm, relaxed, and peaceful as you should from this meditation.

Meditation, if done correctly, causes your mind to be quiet, calm, and peaceful. By activating mind-body mechanisms mediated through your nervous system it can promote the healing of your back.

While many experts insist that meditation be done in an erect sitting posture, I have found that people who cannot sit because of severe back pain can still benefit from meditation when it is done in a lying down position. Keep this fact in mind when you read other books on meditation. Also, there are now special chairs, bolsters, and other aids available to help you keep your back erect and pain free while you meditate if you choose to go this more traditional route. When sitting is out of the question, however, remember that meditation can be done while lying on your back.

A Final Word

You have seen how harmful stress is for your back. Until recently, however, Western medicine virtually ignored the effect of stress on the back. As a consequence, it has failed to solve the escalating epidemic of back pain.

It is extremely important that you recognize that stress in your life can damage your back. By managing stress, you can cure back pain. **If you choose only one thing to do from the Back To Life Program, practice its stress management techniques. They are that powerful and critical in the healing process.**

A word of caution, however. Reading this chapter is not enough. If you don't start applying stress management techniques, nothing will be accomplished. Don't put it off any longer. Do at least 30 minutes of stress management for your back every day. Get personal help if you need to, but get started today. You owe it to yourself! Once you get started, you will find that practicing stress management can be fun and enjoyable. It will also improve your overall health beyond your greatest expectations!

CHAPTER SEVEN

Eating for a Healthy Back

I N THIS CHAPTER ON NUTRITION and your spine, I will show you how you can help heal your back simply by modifying your diet. The territory I'll be covering is rarely touched upon by doctors or even the world's leading back experts.

In all my years of visiting doctors for my back problems, not one of them mentioned anything to me about diet or the type of food I was eating. Today, if you go to doctors for even gastrointestinal problems, very few will ask you what type of food you eat or give you any advice about your diet.

It is a sad fact but true: Doctors understand very little about nutrition and how the food you eat affects your health. This is largely due to the lack of nutritional training in medical schools. Since the turn of the century, there has been little progress in this direction in spite of the public outcry for nutrition courses in the standard medical school curriculum.

Nutrition is a big part of the medicine of the future, and by applying the guidelines covered in this chapter, you will be getting a head start on not only the health and healing of your back, but the health of your entire body as well.

Nutrition and Your Health

Common sense tells you that the old song, "*The knee bone's connected to the thigh bone…*" is correct, especially when it comes to diet and its impact on your body. We know that wholesome foods containing essential nutrients, taken in balanced quantities, nourish and sustain us. The lack of these foods in your diet can contribute to disease, as can the overeating of certain foods. Other dietary substances can be harmful, even in small or moderate amounts.

The relationship between diet and health is well-documented. Deficiencies of specific vitamins, minerals, and trace elements in the diet have been shown to cause a whole host of diseases such as beriberi, pellagra, rickets, scurvy, anemia, hypothyroidism and goiter, osteoporosis, and others. Very few people dispute the relationship that has been discovered between excess fat intake, cholesterol, and heart disease, or sugar and diabetes. Gout, known as "the rich man's disease," is related to a diet of rich foods, high animal protein intake, caffeine, and alcohol. Dietary fats and chemical additives have been implicated in certain cancers, while smoking is known to contribute to lung disease. Alcohol causes cirrhosis of the liver, and there are many other conditions that are believed to be related to diet such as arthritis, psoriasis, gall bladder disease, diverticulitis, colitis, and peptic ulcer, to name but a few.

What about your back? Which foods, beverages, and chemical substances are harmful to your back, and which ones are beneficial? Knowing the difference and following the guidelines in this chapter will greatly improve the health of your back as well as the quality of your life.

The Back To Life Nutritional Guidelines for a Healthy, Pain-Free Spine

The spine is a supersensitive barometer for what's going on in the rest of your body. Problems in other areas of your body often affect your back, especially if you have a history of back problems. For example, when you have a flu with a fever, intense back pain may accompany the illness.

There are also certain well-studied vitamin deficiencies that are known to cause disease in the spine. A long-standing calcium deficiency in the body may show up in your spine as osteoporosis, a weakening of the structures of the bones. A deficiency in vitamin B12 can cause back pain and degeneration of nerve cells in the spinal cord. Vitamin D deficiency can result in rickets, a condition that can cause severe deformities in the spine, especially in childhood.

Clinical evidence suggests that there are other dietary deficiencies, digestive disturbances, and disorders of eating that can have a detrimental effect on your back. In the sections that follow, these problems are addressed with specific, easy-to-follow guidelines to help you establish healthy eating patterns for a pain-free back.

WATCH YOUR WEIGHT

Excess weight affects the spine in a number of ways. First, the sheer weight of a large belly and body pressing on the back muscles and discs causes tension, misalignment, and pain. This creates poor posture, which puts the spine at further risk for injury and strain. Second, it is more difficult for heavy people to get up after sitting down, and to move around in general. As a consequence, there is likely to be less movement in the joints and body. This lack of movement causes the body of an overweight person to be generally much stiffer than that of a normal-weight individual of the same age. The stiffness plus the added weight increases the chances of back strain and injury, and augments whatever pain may be already present. Also, since back pain restricts movement, eating becomes one of the only enjoyable activities left. You eat more and burn fewer calories as your metabolism slows down from a lack of physical activity. Sound familiar?

Since depression of some form usually accompanies prolonged back pain, eating can also be used as a temporary mood elevator. Of course, this short-sighted approach usually backfires, as the increased weight puts more pressure on the back, causing more pain and more depression.

To prevent overeating and excess weight gain, follow these guidelines:

✦ **Avoid fats.** Fat has no fiber, no vitamins, no protein, no carbohydrates for energy, and no taste! As Dean Ornish, M.D., says, "No one raids the oil jar when they get up in the middle of the night!" Try to keep your daily fat intake to 10-20 percent (20-30 grams) per day. This will keep you from gaining weight, which puts pressure on your back.

✦ **Avoid fast foods**, since these are almost always high in fat, low in fiber, low in water, and high in refined sugar and salt. Try to eat three balanced meals each day, including a healthy snack before bed like a piece of fruit. Eat breakfast regularly, since you will need fuel in your body to start your day. Eating breakfast will also keep you from overeating at lunch and dinner.

✦ **Avoid going for long periods of time without food**, since you will become very hungry and more than make up for the meals missed with excess eating.

MAKE SURE YOU GET ENOUGH REST

In this fast-paced world, it is easy for your body to become tired, overworked, sleep-deprived, or worn out and sheer exhaustion results. The obvious remedy for being tired and overworked is rest.

Even though you know that when you are tired you should rest, you usually don't take the time to do it. You tell yourself that you are too busy to afford the luxury of rest. You push on, and take caffeine and other stimulants to help keep yourself awake and functioning after your body's natural energy is depleted. Cocaine and speed have become such popular drugs today because they allow you to function with hyperefficiency, getting all of your work done with minimal rest or sleep. But at what expense?

Fatigue and chronic lack of sleep can have a damaging effect on your back. Your spine needs rest as much, if not more, than any other part of your body. Much of the back pain experienced today is due to overwork and fatigue of not only the back muscles, but the entire body.

Fatigue also creates additional stress in your life. This stress affects the nervous system and the muscles in your back, causing them to tense, tighten, and even spasm. And this causes back pain. Here are a few tips for avoiding sleep deprivation and the stress it creates:

+ Try to get at least 7½-8 hours of sleep every night.

+ Sleep in one day on the weekend if you need to.

+ If you have the time, take an afternoon nap or a siesta for at least 30 minutes.

+ Listen to your body. Listen to your back. To heal, you must be gentle and kind to your body.

+ When you feel tired, rest. Remember, rest is best!

ELIMINATE STIMULANTS

Many people are habituated or addicted to caffeine in the form of coffee, tea, and cola beverages; nicotine, in the form of cigarettes and chewing tobacco; and other stimulants including amphetamines and diet pills.

The extra energy provided by stimulants is borrowed energy from your body's own reserves. Sooner or later, you must pay back this energy, often with interest. What goes up must come down! And this applies to your body's energy. You've heard of the "crashing from speed" syndrome. The same thing happens in varying degrees with other stimulants, including caffeine and nicotine. A person becomes lethargic, drowsy, and may even collapse into a long, stuporous sleep for days at a time after withdrawing from prolonged stimulant usage.

Stimulants of any kind can be very harmful to your back. This is because of their stimulatory effect on your central nervous system, which in turn stimulates the muscles of the spine, causing them to contract and tighten up. Additionally, stimulants exaggerate the stress response, causing you to overreact to situations which might not otherwise upset you. This also takes its toll on your back.

When you take stimulants you are ignoring your body's natural need to slow down and rest. Sooner or later, there will be a breakdown in your system, and this could affect your back.

If you overindulge in caffeine, for example, and push yourself beyond what is healthy for your body, you may trigger painful muscle spasms in your back, so that you will be forced to lie down and rest. Again, as Dr. Bernie Siegel says, "Pain is nature's reset button!" When you lie down and rest, your back can heal.

I've met people who say that caffeine isn't a problem for them. They assure me that it just doesn't affect them; they can drink a cup of coffee right before bed and it won't keep them awake. But many of these people are usually addicted without even knowing it. They may consume up to ten cups of coffee a day and not feel its effects because their body has developed tolerance over the years. Ask these same people to stop consuming caffeine and see what happens. Intense migraine-type headaches, sometimes with nausea and vomiting, almost always occur within several days. That's how powerfully addictive caffeine can be.

Recent medical surveys indicate that many people are chronically sleep-deprived and do not even know it. When they are sleep deprived, people tend to consume large amounts of coffee or other forms of caffeine, in addition to sugar, to perk themselves up and help make it through the day. Doctors, because they work long hours and are on call at nights, are among the greatest offenders.

Many doctors are sleep-deprived and habituated or addicted to coffee. At almost all doctors' conferences, you can find them huddling around the coffee pot, first thing in the morning. Because of this, most doctors don't tell patients that stimulants could be contributing to their back and health problems.

The Caffeine, Nicotine, Alcohol Cycle

Many people who smoke cigarettes or drink coffee or do both, find that by the evening, they are wound up and in need of relaxation. Alcohol fills this need quite nicely. It is a convenient and legal substance that quiets the mind, soothes the nerves, and distances us from our problems. It seems to be a highly effective stress management tool, readily available in the corner liquor store, grocery market, downtown bar, your favorite restaurant, or any social gathering. It's a common part of everyday life.

Alcohol relaxes you because it is a central nervous system depressant, and if you drink enough of it, it can eventually put you to sleep. If you have more than one drink in the evening, you can usually still feel its effects the following morning when it is time to go to work. You feel sluggish, tired, and mentally foggy after an evening of drinking.

To help clear the head and wake you up, a strong cup of freshly-brewed coffee usually does the trick! You can follow this with a second cup of coffee, either at home or the office, and before long, you're feeling pretty good. No matter how tired or out of sorts you felt when you woke up, you're now ready to take on the day! Add a cigarette or two if you are inclined to use nicotine, and you have a chemical formula for a successful morning launch, even after a night of hard drinking!

Since the caffeine and/or nicotine have helped to wake you up and give you a boost, you can continue to have one or both of these substances at regularly-scheduled intervals throughout the day. These chemicals seem to help you do your work more efficiently, keep you from becoming tired or falling asleep, and improve your productivity.

By evening, you might be wound up or completely exhausted after a hard day of work. You might even be a little stressed. Your body may be exhausted, but your mind is reeling with activity following the emotional anxieties of the day.

It is time to wind down, enjoy a relaxing evening and prepare for sleep with a cocktail, beer, or glass of wine. Since one drink makes you feel good, surely one more couldn't hurt! You might have several more before finally going to sleep.

Morning may again find you sluggish, lethargic, and slightly foggy. But a cup of strong coffee or a cigarette will get your juices flowing again. Come evening, you're ready to relax with more alcohol. The cycle continues.

The use of these substances keeps you on an emotional roller coaster all day long. The stimulants speed you up, increasing your response to stress, your mental activity, and your body's production of adrenalin, making it necessary to use alcohol as a sedative to help you calm down come evening. The sedative property of alcohol, which lingers in the morning, is overcome with stimulants such as caffeine and nicotine.

The caffeine, nicotine, and alcohol cycle can persist for years. Since all of these substances are habit-forming, and possibly even addictive, it is difficult to break the cycle once it is established.

Eventually these substances take their toll on the body. Back problems can develop in people who are caught up in this cycle or one of its variations: caffeine and alcohol, nicotine and alcohol, or caffeine and nicotine. Other substances such as tranquilizers, diet pills, prescription drugs, or other over-the-counter medications can be substituted or added to the mix.

If you are currently experiencing problems with your back and are habituated to any of these substances, you may find that if you stop using them, your back will heal immediately.

CHEW YOUR FOOD WELL BEFORE SWALLOWING AND EAT SLOWLY

Inadequate chewing, or mastication, of your food can lead to the production of excess intestinal gas and indigestion. This is usually caused by eating on the run when you are in a hurry, while your mind is engaged in other activities, such as watching television, reading the newspaper, or involved in animated conversation, or when you are upset. Improper attention to the act of eating when you are chewing your food, as basic as this may sound, is responsible for a great many intestinal and digestive problems that can lead to heartburn and gastritis, which causes excess intestinal gas. Due to the proximity of the intestines to the back, the toxins and the pressure from the gas can affect the condition of your back and cause severe back pain.

Here are a few simple tips:

✦ Eat more slowly, chew well, and concentrate on your food. Remember not to eat when you are in a hurry.

✦ Try to remember to sit down when you eat. Make it a point to relax and enjoy your food.

✦ Eating should be a celebration, so give thanks and appreciate your food.

✦ Do not watch television, read the newspaper, or engage in other activities while eating.

Chewing your food well and eating slowly will help prevent gas, improve digestion, and help your back.

ELIMINATE FOODS THAT CAUSE DIGESTIVE PROBLEMS

Certain foods just don't mix well with other foods. This can lead to digestive disturbances which can affect your back.

If you take a glass of lemonade and pour it into a glass of milk, you will see the milk curdle as the lemonade is added, causing a chemical reaction that liberates gases. Now imagine that this is occurring in your stomach. Many food combinations can cause the same chemical reactions in your stomach and intestines.

As part of your body's normal flora, there are over 100 strains of bacteria living at different levels of your intestines. Since they can produce gas as a by-product of their metabolic activity, it is important to know what kinds of foods your body can tolerate, and in what combinations, without forming gas.

Generally, foods or substances that increase the acid production in the stomach and the intestines, or are acidic themselves, tend to produce gas. This includes meats and rich, oily foods. Nuts and beans are also notorious for producing gas. Certain acidic fruit juices, such as orange, grapefruit, and pineapple, as well as vinegar and tomato paste or sauces can also produce gas.

Carbonated drinks produce gas because they have gas in the form of carbon dioxide in their composition. Many people are habituated to the fizz in sodas and soft drinks, not to mention the caffeine, and can consume half a dozen or so during an average day. This adds up to a lot of gas in the system. If you are plagued with back problems and are wondering why, this could be the reason. Try not taking any carbonated drinks for two weeks and see what happens to your back. You may be be pleasantly surprised!

Coffee and tea can be very upsetting to the stomach, intestines and digestive system because they contain caffeine and tannic acid, and stimulate the parietal cells in the stomach to secrete hydrochloric acid. This is especially true when they are taken on an empty stomach. Andrew Weil, M.D., considers coffee to be an intestinal poison for this reason. When I was younger, I drank coffee and I developed an ulcer. I no longer drink it. Even to this day it causes heartburn, gas, and stomach pain if I should have so much as one cup.

Red meat, fowl, and fish are among the hardest of all foods to digest because they are animal proteins. When a baby is learning how to eat solid foods, these proteins are the last to be introduced into the diet because they are so hard to digest. When foods are hard to digest, they remain in the intestines longer. Since animal protein has no fiber and remains in the intestines longer than any other food, it tends to produce foul-smelling gases that can contribute to back problems.

EAT A DIET RICH IN FIBER

Fiber in the diet prevents constipation, which can contribute to the accumulation of toxins in the intestinal tract and the production of gas. Its addition to the diet has been encouraged to help prevent colon cancer and other forms of cancer, as well as heart disease.

Fiber is extremely helpful for people with back problems because of its ability to absorb toxins, reduce intestinal gas, decrease transit time in the intestines, and keep bowel functions regular.

Fiber is not found in animal products (red meat, dairy products, chicken, fish, or other seafoods), nor is it found in processed and refined flours and breads. Because we consume a great deal of these foods in our daily diet, we are falling prey to a whole host of diseases that our ancestors never experienced. The epidemic of back pain that we are now seeing throughout the developed world may in fact be related to a diet high in fat, sugar, and refined flours, and low in fiber, which is so typical of the modern fast foods that most people consume daily.

A diet with adequate fiber consists of fruits and grains for breakfast; raw vegetables, cooked vegetables, and legumes for lunch; vegetables, legumes, and grains or a starchy vegetable like a potato, sweet potato, or squash for dinner; with an after-dinner snack consisting of fruits. Fruits are high in fiber and can also be eaten in between meals as a snack. Dried fruits are also high in fiber, but can be gas-producing if not chewed properly or if taken in excess.

Commercial preparations of fiber are available as additions to regular meals, but it is preferable to take fiber naturally in the foods you eat. Adding fiber artificially to a diet that is high in processed foods and refined flours is usually inadequate. It's like eating junk food and then taking vitamins to compensate instead of getting the vitamins from the foods directly.

DRINK PLENTY OF WATER AND OTHER FLUIDS

Your body is 70 percent water. There is water inside and surrounding the tiniest cells, in the blood, lymph, cerebrospinal fluid, in every organ tissue, in the synovial fluid of your joints, and in the muscles and discs of the spine.

You lose water every day from your body in the breath that is exhaled from your lungs, from the pores in your skin, and from your bowels and bladder. Depending on the climate in which you live, and your level of physical activity, the total amount of water lost each day can vary from 2.5 liters to almost 7 liters. You need to replace this lost water, otherwise you will suffer from dehydration.

Inadequate water intake on a daily basis will affect the health of your spine, since the more water you take into your body, the easier it is to eliminate toxins that might build up through physical activity, stress, chemical additives in the diet, allergy, or low grade infection.

These toxins can accumulate in the bloodstream and nervous system, and make their way to the muscles of your back. It is important to help flush these toxins by replacing the water you lose every day. Whatever water is taken in excess will be eliminated by the kidneys, so it is virtually impossible to consume too much water or fluids in a day.

Adequate fluid intake will aid the process of elimination by both the kidneys and bowels. In the bowels, this will promote the elimination of gases and stools in a timely manner while preventing constipation. Many a case of constipation has been cured by merely adding more water to a diet. As I mentioned earlier, there seems to be a special relationship between the bowels and the back, and improving bowel function can help alleviate back problems. Increasing your daily water intake may be all that's required to help you overcome your back pain.

Certain substances, such as caffeine and alcohol, act as diuretics and can contribute to dehydration in your body by causing excess water to be eliminated through the kidneys. Again, avoid these substances for the sake of your back.

How much water is enough? When your urine is clear like tap water, consider your water intake to be adequate. When your urine is dark yellow, consider your body to be low on fluids. (Certain vitamins can darken the color of your urine, so please take these into account.)

Water, soups, fruit juices, fruits, vegetables, and herbal teas are excellent sources of fluid that can replace the water lost each day from your body.

EAT TWO OR MORE SERVINGS OF VEGETABLES A DAY

Vegetables are good for your back. Studies in the field of international health have shown that cultures that consume the highest amount of vegetables in their diet have the lowest rates of back problems, as well as cancer and heart disease.

Vegetables are an excellent food source since they contain a multitude of beneficial nutrients, including essential vitamins, minerals, trace elements, fiber, water, carbohydrates, and proteins, all of which are required for healthy back muscles and bones.

In nature, the largest animals subsist strictly on vegetables. Elephants, giraffes, hippopotamuses, rhinoceroses, water buffalo, cows, and horses all maintain their huge bodies and large muscle masses by eating only vegetable nutrients, mainly grasses and leaves.

Like these animals, your back also contains large muscles that must be provided with optimal nutrition in order to stay healthy. Vegetables are the best all-around dietary source for this purpose.

Try to have vegetables during at least two meals every day. They can be either cooked or raw, such as a salad with a variety of added vegetable toppings like tomatoes, sprouts, mushrooms, carrots, and so on.

EAT FRUIT AT LEAST TWICE A DAY

The cells in the muscles, tendons, ligaments, nerves, and bones of your spine all require the burning of simple sugars for their metabolism. These sugars provide the essential fuel that the body utilizes to produce energy. Glucose and fructose, the two most common simple sugars found in nature, are both present in fruits and they are rapidly absorbed and taken into the body whenever you eat fruit. In no other foods are these two sugars found together.

Fruits also contain water, essential vitamins, minerals, trace elements, and fiber, all of which are important nutrients for keeping the cells and tissues of your back healthy and strong. Fruits taste great, and when taken in adequate quantities, satisfy your cravings for sugar in the form of candy, processed sweet junk food, or other products with refined sugars, which usually contain empty calories and lack the other health-promoting nutrients so necessary for a strong back.

Fruits can be used for dessert or eaten as healthy snack foods. Because of their high water content, fruits are also excellent sources for replacing the water lost each day from your body. The combination of water and fiber make fruits ideal for helping to regulate bowel function, eliminate toxins from your spine, alleviate gas, and reduce back pain.

EAT A DIET RICH IN WHOLE GRAINS

Whole grains contain a number of beneficial nutrients for your back including protein, fiber, and an abundance of vitamins, minerals, trace elements, and especially carbohydrates, the preferred dietary fuel of athletes, which can provide a steady supply of energy to your spine over a long period of time. Some of the most natural and best sources of fiber come from cooked whole grains, such as brown rice, wheat, oats, barley, millet, corn, rye, and buckwheat. They have traditionally served as the main dietary staple in the majority of the world's populations for thousands of years.

To get optimal nutritional value for your back, stick to whole grain products and flours made from whole grains, which includes whole wheat breads. Try to avoid foods made with white flour, white rice (eat brown rice instead), and other refined grain products since they have been stripped of most of their nutrients and they lack dietary fiber.

EAT BEANS AND LEGUMES FOR PROTEIN
TO NOURISH THE MUSCLES IN YOUR BACK

Proteins are the building blocks for muscles, and since the health of your back depends on healthy muscles, it is important to get at least 2 ounces of protein in your diet every day. The advantages of beans and legumes, including soy products, as sources of protein over animal products are:

+ Beans and legumes contain virtually no fat or cholesterol, whereas animal-derived proteins usually contain high amounts of fat and cholesterol.

+ They help keep your weight down, which will directly benefit your back.

+ They provide more vitamins, minerals, trace elements, and carbohydrates than animal products.

+ Beans and legumes do not contain toxins and other harmful chemicals often found in meats.

Beans and legumes are available in a wide variety of forms. In addition to old-fashioned bean soup and casserole recipes, you can try tofu, seitan, tempeh, as well as delicious meat-substitute products such as burgers, hot dogs, sausage patties, and bacon. These products are completely derived from vegetables, are high in protein, fiber, and other nutrients, and are low in fat.

To further help strengthen the muscles in the back, there are also numerous, low-fat protein powders derived from soy beans that can be conveniently added to bread recipes or fruit smoothies.

Natural Supplements for Your Back

When back pain becomes severe, doctors often prescribe strong anti-inflammatories, muscle relaxants, and narcotic pain medication. However, these medications may have undesirable side effects and can cause additional problems.

If you are seeking gentler, more natural alternatives to these potent and sometimes toxic drugs, there are herbal, plant, mineral, and vitamin remedies that can be effective in alleviating pain and promoting healing.

Because I believe strongly in the benefits of a sound diet, I don't want to give undue emphasis to the use of supplements in treating back pain, even if they are natural. In certain cases, however, I have found them to be effective. A few of the more common natural agents are described here. They are available in different forms, including capsules, tablets, as teas, or as tinctures or extracts. Dosages will depend on the form in which they are taken, as well as your weight, size, and activity level. A pharmacist or health care provider familiar with these products can help you find the dosage that will be safe and effective for you.

Because these substances are generally safer and milder than the stronger drugs, they can often be combined for a synergistic effect. In most cases, they can also be safely added to any current existing conventional medical regimen you may be on. Remember to listen to your body, however. If you develop a rash or any untoward side effects from the introduction of any new substance into your body, it is wise to discontinue the use of that substance.

Here are the natural herbal, vitamin, and mineral supplements I recommend:

+ Valerian Root, in the form of a tea, capsule, or tablet, is an excellent tranquilizer and muscle relaxant without the side effects of stronger medications. Taken in the evening before bed, it can be very effective in promoting sleep, rest, and relaxation of the muscles in the back, and as a natural pain reliever. Since it comes in different forms, precise dosages may vary. A local pharmacist or herbalist can help you. The newer commercial preparations have this information written on the label. Taken as directed, valerian root is safe and effective.

+ Comfrey Root, also in tea, capsule or tablet form, taken 2-3 times daily, stimulates the healing process in injured muscles, tendons, ligaments, bones, and discs. In European folk medicine it is called "knitbone" for its ability to speed the healing process of fractures.

+ Chamomile, most commonly taken as a tea, is also available in capsule or tablet form. It acts on the nervous system as a tranquilizer and in the muscles as a mild relaxant. While it can be taken in the daytime to help soothe the nerves and relax the muscles of the back, it is best taken at night to help alleviate insomnia when the stress and tension of back pain are interfering with a good night's sleep.

+ Cramp Bark, available as a tea, or in capsule or tablet form, is an antispasmodic and muscle relaxant. It is particularly helpful for muscle spasms in the back or when your back is knotted-up, tight, tense, and painful. It can be taken 2-3 times a day. Check dosages with an herbalist or a pharmacist familiar with herbs.

+ Melatonin is a naturally-occurring hormone found in the human body that is produced by the pineal gland. It normalizes circadian rhythms and helps to regulate sleep. Most commercial melatonin is plant-derived, safe, nontoxic, yet highly effective for normalizing sleep and inducing relaxation. It is very effective for people with back pain who cannot sleep at night because of the pain. Average starting dosages range from 1-6 mg taken before bed. You can ask your local pharmacist or herbalist for more specific dosage information that is appropriate for you.

+ Willow Bark contains the compound salicin, which is related to the active ingredient in aspirin, acetylsalicylic acid. It is available in capsules, tablets, or it can be made into a tea. Willow Bark has both anti-inflammatory and pain relieving properties, and for people looking for natural alternatives to the stronger, synthetic drugs prescribed for similar purposes, it can be very helpful. Dosages depend on the form in which it is taken, as well as your weight and activity level.

+ Passion Flower is another useful herb for insomnia, again a common condition for people with back pain. It acts on the nervous system as a mild tranquilizer, muscle relaxant, and pain reliever, and is often found in commercial preparations in combination with Willow Bark or other herbs whose activity is similar. It is most commonly found as a tea but is also available as a capsule, tablet, or tincture.

+ Bromelain is a naturally-occurring enzyme found in pineapples. In certain cases it may help inflammation and swelling in the back, particularly around the discs. Formerly, in large medical centers, it was routinely injected directly into the discs to reduce the symptoms of disc herniation and rupture. Taken orally, it may help diminish your back pain.

+ Arnica is a plant that is relied upon in homeopathy for the treatment of joint disease and back pain. It can be taken internally in homeopathically-produced form, or as a topical gel rubbed into the area of inflammation and pain. It is a very effective agent in reducing inflammation and pain while stimulating the healing process.

+ St. John's Wort is highly effective in the management of chronic pain and the depression that usually accompanies pain. It is available in commercially-prepared capsules and tablets, as well as in dried bulk for teas. Because of its potency, it is recommended that you not take it if you are currently taking other conventional antidepressant medication.

+ Vitamin C is a cofactor in wound healing. It aids in the repair of damaged tissues such as muscle, tendon, bone, and ligament. Well-known author Norman Cousins used vitamin C along with laughter to help him overcome a terminal arthritic illness of the spine known as Ankylosing Spondylitis. Vitamin C is available in citrus fruits and juices, and many other fruits and vegetables. It also can be taken safely as an extract. The average maximum adult dosage is 2-4 grams per day, but it may be too acidic for your stomach, so take it with plenty of fluids or a little food. Again, check with your pharmacist, herbalist, or physician for the appropriate dosage for you.

+ Other vitamins, minerals, and trace elements are also helpful in overcoming back pain and promoting a healthy, strong spine. Daily dosages vary depending on the individual, so please check with your pharmacist or a nutritionist for doses appropriate for you:

  + Boron helps build strong bones.

  + Vitamin B complex helps build strong and healthy bones and muscles in the back.

  + Vitamin E, as an antioxidant, helps to repair damaged muscle tissue in the back.

  + Magnesium builds strong bones while helping the muscles in the back contract and relax.

  + Selenium helps build strong bones and muscles in the back.

+ Numerous topical herbal pain balms are also available. They create heat, dilate blood vessels, improve blood flow where applied, and are very soothing and effective for relieving back pain from tired, sore, achy muscles. Tiger Balm is probably the best known pain balm in this category, but there are many others that usually include capsicum and menthol as their main ingredients. Pain balms are very effective when applied at night before sleep, and because they create heat in the back, are also effective at times when the back is susceptible to chilling, such as in winter weather.

A Final Word

Your body is not a machine or an inanimate object, but rather a living, breathing, dynamic organism. In order to grow, repair itself, and remain healthy, it needs good food. Because everything you eat gets broken down into chemicals that affect the health of the tiniest cell in your body including the muscle cells, nerve cells, bone cells, and ligament cells that make up the tissues in your back, you must be aware of what you put into your mouth and what effect it will have on your back.

You owe it to yourself to be conscious of how and what you eat. If you want your back to heal and become strong and healthy, follow the Back To Life nutritional guidelines presented in this chapter. If you would like further information on this subject, please refer to the recommended reading list in the Appendix.

CHAPTER EIGHT

Back To Work:
Slow and Steady Wins the Race

THINKING ABOUT GOING BACK TO WORK after a painful back injury or strain can be frightening. Because of the powerful influence the mind has on the body, these fearful thoughts alone can produce the kind of anxiety and stress that will increase your back pain and worsen your condition, making a timely return to work seem even more remote.

In this chapter, you will learn how to ease yourself back into your work routine and take care of your back so it becomes stronger and better able to withstand the physical and mental stresses of your job.

Returning To Work as Soon as Possible

The day before I was supposed to report to the Air Force to begin my four year tour of duty, my back went out in a very painful way. I reported to the orthopedic surgeon for an evaluation of my spine with the hope that he would write me a medical waiver and I could delay reporting for military duty. After a cursory exam, he determined that there was no permanent structural damage in my back, and he blatantly asked, "Are you afraid of entering the military?"

I defiantly answered, "No, I'm not." But underneath my assertiveness, I was. With my conscious mind trying its best to suppress my fear, the truth of the matter was that I wasn't exactly looking forward to my upcoming military duty. Would I be sent off to war? Would I get shot? Would I get thrown in the federal penitentiary for accidentally breaking some military rule or regulation?

While I tried to put these thoughts out of my mind, they weighed heavily on my back, creating stress and tension. The result was incapacitating pain that delayed the start of my military career by a full five months.

At another time in my life, following my painful back operation and after I had completed military service, the thought of going back to work sent spasms into the muscles of my spine. I was in a lot of pain and the pain was exhausting me; how could I possibly work? Also, I was worried that my back would go out on me again. I had plunged into one of the darkest periods of my life. Because I was depressed, I didn't want to face anybody. I wanted to be alone, crawl into a hole, and die. The more reclusive I became, however, the more the lack of confidence in my back and myself seemed to grow.

When you are thinking about returning to work, the thought of your back going out on the job, or not getting back to work on time, can actually contribute to making your back worse. In fact, when your back pain first starts to really interfere with your ability to function on a day-to-day basis, just the thought of not being able to work and all that that implies, including missed paychecks, unpaid bills, overdue rent, mortgages, and so on, can interfere with your back's ability to heal itself. These thoughts, based on fear, create more tension and stress, tightening your back muscles while increasing your pain. This produces more fear and pain, creating a dangerous cycle.

Sometimes the best way to overcome your fear is to face it head on and return to work as soon as possible, even if only part-time or while performing light duties. For the sake of healing your back, it is much better to do this than to lie at home feeling sorry for yourself and lamenting over the possibility that you will never be able to work again.

At my tenth annual medical school class reunion, one of my colleagues, who was an orthopedic surgeon, shared data from studies that proved conclusively that the most important thing for someone suffering from chronic back pain is to return to work as soon as possible. It helps keep their mind off problems, gives them an opportunity to interact with other people, improves self-esteem through earning money and contributing to their family's welfare, and makes them feel more valuable as a human being. It actually aids the overall healing process.

The more you stew about your back and your inability to meet the challenge of your work, the more stress you'll create for yourself and the worse your back will get. The sooner you get back to work, the faster your back will heal.

Having said that, however, you don't want to completely ignore your back pain by popping painkillers and continuing to work when your back needs to rest. This will interfere with the healing process and make your back worse. You could end up on an operating table like I did because I just wouldn't leave my back alone and let it heal in its own time. Even after my operation, I didn't let my back heal. I took painkillers and pressed on, working from early morning until late into the night, including weekends, and running around like a fool. Don't be stupid like me.

Easing Back into the Work Routine

The best way to get back into the work routine is by testing the waters with your back. See if your doctor will write you a note recommending light duties or part-time work. When you return to your job, work only half days for the first two weeks. This will help you gradually adjust to the hustle and bustle of the work environment without pushing yourself beyond your limits.

In Japanese Zen Buddhism, there is a metaphor about the bamboo plant that might help you remember not to push your back beyond its capacity when you are preparing to return to work. The bamboo is the strongest wood in the world for its weight and size. In the Orient and throughout Asia, wherever bamboo grows, huge skyscrapers are built with workers standing on scaffolding that has been erected with bamboo poles lashed together with rope. These bamboo scaffolds often extend more than 20 stories high.

Bamboo is mostly hollow. When it grows, it grows in sections. After growing a certain length, the bamboo plant will form a horizontal plate, like a joint, before the next length of wood is added on. This serves to stabilize and brace the wood, allowing section upon section to be added until the plant is very tall. Bamboo poles are known for their incredible strength and lightness for this reason. The key is in the horizontal plate. As it grows, bamboo knows to take support before adding the next segment to its height. In other words, the bamboo's true strength lies in the wisdom of knowing its own limitations.

When you return to work, you may find it helpful to keep this image of the bamboo in mind. The more you respect your back's limitations, the stronger your back will grow.

Your ability to work at full capacity depends on how much confidence you have in your back. If you are insecure about your back's ability to hold up at work, your fear will cause your back to tighten up and, most likely, you will slip back into the pain-fear-tension cycle.

Increase your self-confidence and make your back stronger by understanding where your back pain is coming from, learning to listen to your body, becoming more familiar with the way your back works and how it is connected to the rest of your body, and by practicing techniques of stress management, stretching, and strengthening (see Chapters Five and Six).

In addition, to take better care of your back as it performs for you at work, follow the suggestions in this chapter and apply them based on your job-specific demands.

How to Make Standing at Work Easier

If you must stand for long periods of time at work, and this causes discomfort for your back, there are several things you can do that are likely to help:

1. Develop good posture. This will help take weight off your back by distributing it evenly over your spine, hips, legs, and feet. Most people are unaware of their posture when they stand, and by increasing awareness, you can often correct imbalances that affect your back (see Chapters Four and Five).

2. Strengthen the muscles in your calves and thighs. This will also help make it easier to stand since stronger legs will help take the burden off your back when you are standing, lifting, and carrying heavy objects (see Chapter Five).

3. As you stand, slowly shift the weight of your body from one leg to the other. Notice which side feels better. Many people unconsciously bear a majority of their weight on one side of the body when standing, usually the dominant side. For example, right-handed people often place more weight on the right leg, right foot, and right side of the body, and this is often the side where they have back pain. Become aware of how you stand and how the weight of your body is distributed over your feet. Experiment with different positions of your feet and legs. For example, if you are used to standing with your feet together, try standing with your feet a little wider apart. Try arching your back gently with your knees slightly bent.

4. The standing poses in yoga (see Chapter Four and the Appendix) will help build strength, stamina, and balance in your feet, legs, hips, and back, making it easier for you to stand for longer and longer periods. Tai Chi, a popular and gentle martial art from China, involves the practice of standing in a variety of positions and it can be very helpful for people with back problems. If Tai Chi classes are available in your area, I urge you to enroll. The time spent will be well worth it.

5. The type of shoe you wear and the sole on the bottom of your shoe will make a big difference to the health of your back when you

stand. A well-supported, wide-based, firm, yet forgiving sole that will help absorb the shocks of standing and walking—like those found in walking and other athletic shoes—will reduce the forces transferred upward to the back. There are also shoe inserts designed to reduce the impact on the spine.

6. The type of surface you stand on will also make a difference to the health of your back. Concrete floors are the hardest on the feet and back because they have no give. They can put a strain on the muscles, bones, and joints, especially after many hours. Wooden floors or carpeted floors are better. Special mats and padding for hard surfaces are now available to help overcome muscle fatigue and pain in the legs and back. If these are not already in place at work, ask for them.

7. If you find yourself standing for prolonged periods, it will also help your back if you lean up against a wall, table, countertop, or high-backed chair whenever possible. Remember to take support as often as you can, just like the bamboo.

8. Sitting down periodically after prolonged standing will help take the load off your back and rest the muscles of the lower extremities. It is important to sit with good posture in a way that doesn't put undue pressure on your discs.

Why Walking on the Job Will Strengthen Your Back

Walking is one of the most important activities you can do for your health; it is the best and safest form of exercise. The more you can walk on the job, the less you will have to schedule time for it outside of work, and the healthier you will be at the end of each day. You don't see door-to-door mail carriers scheduling time for exercise after work, and as a rule, they are an extremely healthy group.

Walking is good medicine. We know it is good for the heart, it increases circulation, and it is gentle on the joints. Even people with arthritis can benefit from walking. In fact, both the American Heart Association and the National Arthritis Foundation recommend that we all walk a minimum of 30 minutes per day, 3-6 days a week to improve our health.

Walking is good for your mental and emotional health as well; studies have shown that the simple act of walking is extremely effective for relieving stress and tension. By taking your mind off your problems, both your mind and body can relax as you exercise. Walking is now recommended as a primary treatment for people with depression for this very reason.

Almost every job entails a certain amount of walking. Some jobs require more than others. Of course, in this age of automation and hurried time schedules, people find excuses not to walk. Even though we know that walking is good for us, most of us ride elevators or escalators instead of climbing stairs, or we drive around and around in our cars looking for a parking place that will save us from walking a few extra steps.

While walking is good for your heart and mind, it may be even more important for your back, especially if you are practicing good posture while you are walking. It helps develop strength in both your legs and back muscles. Many patients who have back pain while standing or sitting, report that when they walk, they have no pain at all.

Here are a few tips for getting the most out of walking:

✦ When you find yourself walking at work, even a short distance, try to be conscious of each step you take and notice how your back feels.

✦ Experiment with your stride and the placement of your feet, breathing as you walk. See if you tend to place more weight on one foot or one side of the body than the other, which will cause back strain. Adjust your stride, lengthening or shortening it so your back feels comfortable when you walk.

+ Slow down your pace so you can feel how the placement of your feet and the movement of your legs and hips affect the muscles in your spine.

+ Learn to walk in a balanced way that places the least amount of burden on your spine. Try to walk in a gliding, smooth, and fluid motion, and learn to walk and move with your back at the center of your awareness.

+ Feel the connectedness between your back and your legs, thighs, calves, feet, and the rest of your body as you walk. Listen to your body. Discover which muscles feel weak and which muscles feel tight. Take mental notes and then concentrate on strengthening and stretching these muscles according to the guidelines in Chapters Four and Five.

+ Practice walking until you find a rhythm and gait that feels good for your back. It may take a little time and some experimenting.

+ Try to walk without carrying anything at first.

+ Remember to rest if you are walking for long distances.

+ Don't overdo it, but walk as much as you can as often as you can. If you do, you will find your back will become healthy and strong.

Proper Carrying and Lifting for Your Back

Carrying and lifting heavy objects puts an obvious strain on your back. **When you are first returning to work, avoid lifting of any kind for the first two weeks, period.** It will be hard enough sitting, standing, walking, and making it through the day as you get your confidence back.

Follow these simple guidelines for carrying and lifting:

+ When you do begin to lift and carry things, build confidence by starting out with light objects. Build up slowly, adding 5 pounds each week. Slow but steady wins the race.

+ Some objects aren't heavy, but are extremely awkward to carry because of their shape. Be very careful with these. **Always remember to ask for help if something doesn't feel right for you. Know your limitations and exercise caution.** Remember, you can build up slowly. Try not to put your back in a compromising position.

+ Carry objects close to your body, maintaining good posture while letting your legs absorb most of the weight since your leg muscles are your strongest and largest muscles. Let your legs do the lion's share of the work. Walk slowly and deliberately.

+ **Carry less weight and make more trips.** If you have many objects to carry from one place to the next, such as when you are unloading a truck or a moving van, there is a tendency to carry heavier loads to make fewer trips. When I used to help friends move to a new apartment, or when I loaded and unloaded semi-trucks, stacking heavy stereo speakers in the warehouse where I worked, I would always try to maximize my loads to minimize the number of trips I had to make. This was just plain stupid and it caused my back a lot of damage over the years.

   After going through back surgery and being unable to work for three years, I now make as many trips as I need to, knowing that each trip is making my legs and heart that much stronger and ultimately enhancing the quality of my overall health, helping my back in the process.

When lifting, use levers and other aids to bring the object you are lifting high enough so that you don't have to bend down to pick it up. Many injuries occur when you are bending over, since in this position, maximum pressure is placed on the discs of your spine. Add a heavy or awkward weight, and you are placing your spine in the most vulnerable position possible.

If someone handed you 50 pounds while you were already standing erect, and you kept that object close to your body, you could probably carry that weight ¼ mile or more without any strain on your back. Most likely your legs would be aching and would give out first. That same weight, however, if you had to bend over and pick it up from the floor, could do your back in. It's all in the physics and mechanics of the spine.

Many back care manuals, books, and instructional videos make a case out of proper techniques for bending down to pick up a heavy object. Most glorify the "bent-knee" position, keeping the back straight as you use your legs to do the lifting. They recommend that you not pick up anything by bending over with your knees straight.

In theory they are right, but since most of us were not trained to bend our knees and use our legs to do lifting, I find this technique a little awkward and often impractical. It is true that if you bend your knees and keep your back straight while stooping down to pick up an object, you will be better off for it. But I personally feel it is preferable and safer to apply the stretching and strengthening principles we discussed earlier (see Chapters Four and Five). They are:

1. Move slowly and gradually.

2. Avoid jerking.

3. Don't force or strain.

4. Focus on your breathing, exhaling as you lift the object.

5. Don't lift anything by yourself that doesn't feel right for your back.

6. Don't be in a hurry when you lift. Slow but steady wins the race.

Your strength is knowing your limitations. Listen to your body. Remember the story of bamboo. If you are constantly aware of these factors, your abilities will be slowly expanded. Before you know it, you'll be moving pianos like a pro.

Bending Down

Bending down can jeopardize the stability of your spine if it is done suddenly and too soon after a major injury, strain, or operation. Generally, I ask my patients to focus on the stretching and stress management techniques in Chapters Four and Six for at least the first two months following a major spine event while avoiding bending down or other forward-bending movements of the spine.

Because bending down can be a wonderful opportunity to stretch the hamstrings in the back of your thighs, as well as the muscles in the lower lumbar area, you don't want to avoid it forever. If your back feels better after several months, you can test the waters by slowly starting to bend forward again. If you experience pain or discomfort at any time during this process, you must straighten your spine, or if you are unable to do this, drop down on all fours and rest.

When you begin to practice bending down, stand next to a table-top, chair, wall, or desk for support in case you need it. Then follow these steps:

FIRST STAGE: BENDING DOWN

1. Keep your feet shoulder-width apart.

2. As you start to bend down, roll your shoulders forward, then lower your head, neck, and upper body, bending forward at the waist and hips. Remember to move slowly and breathe as you move.

3. Place your hands on your thighs or knees for support. Breathe deeply and relax your spine.

4. Slowly walk your hands down your legs, bending slightly at your knees. In the beginning, bring your hands only as far as your knees if you are able, and then come back up. Over several weeks, gradually increase the distance until you are eventually able to bring your hands down to your shins or ankles.

5. To get back up, inhale slowly and walk your hands and arms back up your legs, using your back and abdominal muscles until you reach an upright position.

   Note: Getting up from a bent-over position puts a lot of pressure on the discs and stresses the muscles in the lower spine, so this must be done slowly, consciously, and with breathing. Remember to place your hands on your legs for support if needed, walking them up the front of your legs as you straighten up.

6. When you've reached an upright position, place your fists in the small of your back and gently bend backward to counter the forward bending movement. Then relax.

SECOND STAGE: BENDING DOWN

Once you've mastered the first stage without any discomfort or pain, try doing the exact same movement without using the help of your arms or hands. Rely solely on the muscles in your back and abdomen to lower and raise your upper body.

1. Stand with your feet slightly apart and your arms relaxed at your sides.

2. As you roll your shoulders forward and lower your upper body, bend

forward at the waist. Tighten your abdominal muscles as you bend forward to help support your back. Keep your arms relaxed by your sides, lowering your upper body only as far as is comfortable.

Note: If you experience discomfort in your back at any time, place your hands and arms on your legs to help brace your back as you did in the first stage. If you get stuck and cannot get back up, simply drop to your hands and knees and rest. Breathe and relax in this position until the pain or discomfort subsides.

3. When you've lowered your upper body as far as is comfortable, relax the muscles in your spine and breathe deeply. Feel the muscles in your lower spine and backs of your legs (hamstrings) stretching. Relax and let gravity do the work, and remember not to force or strain.

4. When you're ready to come up, inhale, and slowly roll your spine up until you've reached an upright position.

5. Place your fists in the middle of your lower back and gently arch your back before returning to a normal standing position.

Sitting at Work

Sitting puts tremendous pressure on the discs, particularly if proper posture is not maintained. This is why most back pain sufferers find sitting to be the most painful of all activities. While sitting can be helpful to give your legs a rest after prolonged standing, it is important to sit with good posture and support for your back. Most of us have not been taught how to sit properly.

A lumbar support or a chair that is designed to take the weight off the spine (see Appendix) will maintain a proper concave, lordotic curve in the lower spine (see Chapter Two, page 21). This shifts the weight off the discs and back onto the rear portions of the bony vertebrae. With proper posture, you can sit for much longer periods of time and when you get up, you'll feel much better.

For prolonged sitting, try to avoid backless stools and chairs, as well as soft-cushioned sofas and comfort chairs that offer little support. Your back likes firm support to help keep it aligned and the muscles toned. The same principle applies to mattresses. When they are too soft, there is no support for the muscles or bones in your spine and back pain can be made much worse.

Try not to sit for more than 30 minutes at a stretch. If you are just returning to work after a significant back strain, injury, or an operation on your back, you may want to get up, stretch the muscles in your back and legs, walk around, and re-establish proper posture by gently extending and stretching your spine for at least five minutes every half hour. Since sitting favors the forces of flexion and compression of your spine, you can open and improve your posture through gentle back-bending, extending your spine when you stand up, or even while sitting. If you work at a computer terminal or desk, it is important to do extension stretches at regular intervals throughout your day, since the forces of flexion over time will mold and compress your back into a bent over position that places you at greater risk for more back problems.

A wonderful sitting position for the back is the Japanese squatting pose (see Chapter Four). Try sitting on the soles of your feet with your knees bent, like the Japanese do when eating or drinking tea. This position takes all the pressure off your spine and helps to stretch the muscles in your hips, pelvic area, and lower spine. It requires fairly flexible knees and a soft, cushioned surface to kneel on. You can also try placing pillows or folded blankets behind your knees. There are several back chairs on the market that are designed to accommodate this posture. I am sitting on one right now as I write these words on my computer.

Getting Up from a Seated or Lying Down Position

Getting up from a seated position requires strong legs. If your legs are weak, then you need strong arms. If both your arms and legs are weak, all of the burden of getting up is placed on your back and stomach muscles.

If you are suffering from back pain or have a weak back, getting up from either a sitting or lying down position can have a critical effect on you both mentally and physically. The pain you experience can be particularly demoralizing, especially if it comes on abruptly and catches you by surprise.

To prevent pain from catching you by surprise when you try to get up, focus on strengthening the muscles in your legs and other parts of your body that affect your spine such as your abdominal muscles. The stronger your legs, stomach, and back, the easier it will be to get up without pain. Practice getting up from both a lying down and seated position in a way that doesn't cause pain. Listen to your body. Remember to do the stretching and strengthening exercises in Chapters Four and Five. The more you practice, the easier it will get.

Driving

Truck drivers, heavy equipment operators, bus drivers, taxi drivers, traveling salespeople, and other professionals who must take to the road to earn a living have a high incidence of back problems. This may be due in part to the stresses of driving itself, but it is also a result of the mechanics of prolonged sitting. Sitting for long periods of time is hard on the spine because of increased pressure on the discs and the inability to strengthen or tone your back muscles while in this position.

Sitting at the wheel of any vehicle is virtually a passive activity as far as the muscles of the back are concerned, and they can atrophy from lack of use.

It is important to maintain good posture while driving. Lumbar supports and back cushions in a variety of shapes and sizes are now available in mail order catalogues (see Appendix) and most automotive sections at major department stores and automotive centers. Also, adjustable back supports are now built into the seats of some new cars; some even have sophisticated orthopedic devices to support, heat, and massage the back.

The same principles of spine mechanics that apply to sitting also apply to driving. For long distance drives, try to get out of your vehicle every hour or two and stretch for five minutes. If your schedule won't allow you to take time out from driving, try to stretch as you drive, keeping your eyes on the road and your hands on the wheel. Here's an example of one of the many stretches that can be done while driving:

DRIVING BACK-ARCH STRETCH

+ Breathe deeply and arch your spine, protruding your abdomen to increase the curvature in your lower spine. Pull your shoulders back, stretch your upper back, and expand your chest.

+ As you breathe out, gently contract the muscles in your abdomen, tucking in your tummy, flattening the curve in your lower back, and drawing your shoulders forward.

+ Repeat this movement slowly, alternately arching and flattening your lower back and rolling your shoulders back and forth for several minutes every hour.

Also, try not to let the stress of driving affect you. When you find yourself losing your temper at other people on the road because they are going too slowly and you are afraid you'll be late for work or an important meeting, remember that these stressful feelings are affecting your back. You must try to relax, breathe, and be aware of your back and how it feels. A tense driving experience can really take its toll on your back.

Practice the art of relaxation and do not get bent out of shape (literally) because you are worried that you will be late to your destination. It is better to be late, but safe and sound, relaxed, and pain-free, with your peace of mind and spine intact.

Airline Travel on the Job

If you spend a lot of time flying, airline travel can be stressful and exhausting. Time zone changes, cramped sitting positions, inferior food and air quality, as well as unnatural temperature changes all take their toll on your back.

Being away from home, sleeping in strange beds, often with mattresses that are too soft and don't offer support for the spine, add to the challenge. Here are a few simple guidelines:

+ For long airline trips, request an aisle seat so that you can get up frequently and walk the aisles or stretch in the back section, taking a load off your spine.

+ If you can afford it, choose a first class or business class seat, which are roomier and easier on the spine. If you can't, remember to bring a lumbar support for your lower spine and to dress comfortably, preferably wearing clothes that are loose fitting so that you can stretch and move around in them.

+ Check as much luggage as you can so you aren't burdened with heavy carry-on bags that you have to tote around with you. When you get to the airport and have heavy bags, it's cheaper to spend $5-$10 on a porter who can check your bags all the way through to your final destination than it is to spend $2,000 a night in the hospital and be out of work for two weeks to a month. Again, the key is learning to ask for help and also learning to be good to yourself and your back, even if it costs a little more. You're definitely worth it!

+ At hotels, the same guidelines apply. Be good to your back. Let the bellman take your bags. Request a firm bed. See if they'll let you test the mattress before you check in. If all the mattresses are soft, request a board to be placed beneath the mattress to firm it up. Because back problems are so widespread, almost all hotels will be prepared to accommodate you.

During my military assignments, and when I used to travel to medical conferences, I slept on the floors of the fanciest hotels since the soft mattresses made my back feel worse and the firmness of the floor felt good for my back while it was still recovering from surgery. The housecleaning crew would arrive in the mornings to find the bedsheets, pillows, and blankets all on the floor! I'm sure it must have seemed peculiar to them that a person would pay so much money just to sleep on the floor!

Helping Your Back by Asking for Help

For most of us with back problems the hardest thing to do is to ask for help. Why? Perhaps our pride is at stake. Perhaps on a subconscious level we think we should be able to handle our responsibilities alone, and since we want to be independent, we need to learn to fend for ourselves. Perhaps we think we are not worthy of help, that other people are more important than we are and that they have more important things to do than to help us.

Our inability to ask for help may stem from deep-seated feelings of inadequacy. "Who are we to ask for help?" we may ask. We think we have to bear the entire burden of life and the problems of the world on our own shoulders.

Whatever the reasons, I have noticed this peculiar inability to ask for help in myself and in many patients I have treated over the years. But asking for help is one of the most significant lessons our backs can teach us about life. Contrary to what we've been taught, it is not a sign of weakness, but rather a sign of strength to ask for help when you need it. Once I learned this priceless lesson, my back began to improve.

If you take pride in what you do, you probably tend to follow the axiom, If you want something done right, do it yourself! This is what most of us have been taught, right? I don't disagree with this philosophy. However, when it comes to your back, it's just not healthy for you to do everything by yourself all the time. To reduce the workload and strain on your back, it is necessary for you to speak up for yourself and ask for help when it is needed.

Practicing the art of asking for help—and it does take practice—is one of the single most important things you can learn to do for your back. The more you practice it, the easier it becomes. The surprising thing is that people will often respond in a warm and friendly manner when you ask for help; it can give you a feeling of being connected to others.

Helping Your Back by Delegating Responsibility

In the military, I was continually reminded that as an officer, one of the most important leadership skills I could learn was how to delegate responsibility to others. This is not as easy as it sounds. When it comes to your back and your work, however, you must learn to do it. The more you are able to delegate to others, the less of a load you will be placing on your back.

Andrew Carnegie, the great steel magnate, and one of the wealthiest men in the history of the world, is said to have known nothing about steel when he started out in his business. He assembled a team of experts, including scientists and businessmen, who met everyday and actually ran the day-to-day affairs of the company. "What was Carnegie's role?" you may ask. He said his role was to make sure everyone got along so the work could go on smoothly! Carnegie knew how to delegate responsibility.

If you are not delegating responsibility, you are probably making things harder on yourself and your back than they have to be. Remember that your back is a sensitive barometer not only for what's going on in your body, but more important, in your entire life. Any forcing or straining that you are doing in any aspect of your life will take its toll on your back.

Your body has a built-in wisdom, and it will use pain and illness as a way of telling you to restore balance to your life. If you have back problems, your back can be the point of initiation into the deeper wisdom of your body.

Don't Be a Workaholic:
Take Time to Smell the Flowers

Many of us define ourselves through our work. Who we are is what we do. We measure our success and achievement as human beings by what we have accomplished in the workplace.

I enjoy working and I certainly don't want to belittle the value of work, but work must be balanced with family, friends, and taking the time to celebrate the joy of life. Otherwise it's over too soon and we miss what life is all about.

If you keep your nose to the grindstone your entire life without taking the time to slow down and smell the roses, by the time you finally do wake up and realize that life is short, you may be too old, feeble, and sickly to enjoy what little time remains for you.

Many people use work as an escape from their personal problems. If things aren't going right in their relationships or personal life, they go to the office and work harder, burying their personal problems in their work. They may think that the harder they work, the more successful they'll become, and soon, all of their problems will be solved. Unfortunately, it rarely turns out this way.

Relationships and personal growth are never easy and they often come at the cost of great pain, but workaholism is not the proper antidote. Workaholism is a dangerous addiction that keeps us from growing emotionally and spiritually as whole people.

If your back is in severe pain at this very moment, this could be your body's way of getting you to slow down and listen. Don't fight it. There's usually an extremely valuable lesson in the pain. The greater the pain, the greater the lesson. Perhaps it has been a long time since you've smelled the flowers.

If things aren't going right at home, don't charge into work to ease the pain. Slow down, take a deep breath, and take a day off to reflect on who you are and what you want for yourself in this life. Treat yourself to a day of fun; you deserve it. Having fun can be therapeutic.

A Final Word

Whatever you do in life, it is important to listen to your body. If your back is continually getting sprained or injured on the job, it may be time for a career or a position change if you can't find a healthier way to do what you are currently doing. If physical abuse is not the problem, but on-the-job mental stress is, your body may be trying to tell you something here as well.

Whatever work you are currently doing, or whatever you aspire to do, when your back is healthy and strong, you stand a much greater chance of excelling and succeeding than if you are injured, crippled, or in pain. As your best friend and life partner, your body is a wise and reliable consultant. To help you make the right choices on the job and with your career, you must learn to listen to and consult with your body.

CHAPTER NINE

Back To Play:
An Essential Ingredient for Healing

A WISE SAGE FROM INDIA once said, "Seriousness is a disease more dangerous than cancer." Research studies are proving that this is true. Your state of mind can affect your immune system to the point where you are at an increased risk for cancer, heart disease, and other life-threatening chronic illnesses if you have little joy, laughter, and fun in your life. This is certainly true of back problems as well.

Many people who have back problems are often afraid to get involved in fun activities they enjoy for fear of reinjury or pain. This is especially true with favorite sports like tennis, skiing, golf, and backpacking, where physical stresses and strains can affect the back. But even if you have severe back problems, you can and must play. It is a critical ingredient in the healing process.

In this chapter, you will learn how to incorporate play into your life, and use it as an essential element in the healing of your back.

Playing and Healing

Play is more of a state of mind, an attitude, than a specific activity. It is doing something for the sake of having fun and for no other reason.

The most important benefit of play is that it focuses your mind on the present moment. When you're not thinking about mistakes of the past or worrying about the future, you can be carefree and relaxed. When you're relaxed, the reduced neurological input from the brain allows the muscles of your back to relax, and this contributes to your healing.

Dr. Bernie Siegel reminds us that in order to heal ourselves from illness, even such serious afflictions as cancer, we must get back to doing the things we enjoyed as children, and in this way achieve the relaxed, stress-free state of mind necessary for true healing to take place. The same is true for your back.

As you think about the many activities you enjoyed as a child, or those you would love to do now if you had the chance, remember that it is the attitude behind the activity, more than the activity itself, that defines a spirit of play. This playful attitude is essential for the health and well being of your back.

Keeping in mind the therapeutic nature of play and how it can benefit your back, here are some activities and ideas that can help you cultivate a spirit of playfulness in your life.

HOBBIES

Hobbies are very important for people with back problems. They help to focus and quiet your mind, which relaxes the muscles in the spine. This relaxation helps eliminate back pain while activating the healing process.

Hobbies calm you down and bring you into that focused state of awareness that happens when you are playing. When you are doing what you love to do, you forget about time. You are neither thinking about the past nor concerned about the future. You are fully absorbed in the present moment, and in this state of awareness, the mind and body are completely relaxed and healing can occur.

Hobbies are very personal. You may have your own hobby that is unique to your particular skills and tastes. My hobbies include music, lapidary, hiking, camping, surfing, gardening, landscaping, writing, traveling, and yoga. Even though I am a busy doctor, I try to stay involved with my hobbies as much as possible.

VACATIONS

Vacations are essential to help relieve stress and excess pressure that gets built up in your system. You must take vacations to maintain your general health and the health of your back. In addition, vacations improve morale and productivity. This is why every company pays their employees to take vacations.

When you take a vacation, it is with the intention of relaxing and getting away from your problems and daily routine through a change of environment. You usually spend a lot of money, time, and preparation, and often travel great distances so that you will have an enjoyable, memorable time.

However, I have seen people stressed on their vacations because either they are taking their problems with them or they are so used to high-speed activity that they can't seem to slow down long enough to relax and enjoy themselves. These people usually have maps and a million-and-one places to go in a very short time, and they tend to run themselves all over and end up getting sick. This is ridiculous because it defeats the purpose of their vacation.

Here are a few tips for a healthy, successful, well-rounded vacation:

✦ Don't plan too much. Be flexible and leave room for spontaneity.

✦ Leave your problems at home and set your mind on automatic pilot as you focus on things that are fun and meaningful to you, taking each day as it comes.

✦ Set aside your worries, obligations, and guilt, and concentrate on doing simple things that help you forget about time.

✦ Try to leave your watch behind. Enter into the timeless state you were in when you were a child, when you had no responsibilities and no pressured engagements to attend. If done right, vacations can be healing experiences. That's why you feel rested, refreshed and renewed when you come back home from a great vacation.

✦ When you are back home in your daily routine, try to remember how you were on vacation. Bring back that relaxed, carefree state of mind as you move through your activities.

✦ Even if you are busy and can't take the time off to travel, practice the art of taking mini-vacations on a daily basis. Close your eyes, relax, and imagine yourself having fun somewhere. Breathe deeply and allow yourself the pleasure of reliving the good times, even if just for a moment.

✦ At least once a week, try to do something or go someplace different. It needn't be far away from your home. Change your perspective. Get outside of yourself. Don't allow yourself to get stuck in a rut or bogged down with drudgery. You can have a vacation when you change your state of mind irrespective of the geography. You needn't journey to some exotic locale to experience the therapeutic benefits of a vacation.

✦ At work, don't bank your vacation time, trading it in for money. Because they can be healing, vacations are more valuable than money.

Your health is a priceless commodity. Take your vacations however you can experience them, and know that by taking a vacation you're making a decision to improve the quality of your health and your life.

ENTERTAINMENT

Entertainment is something done for the pure sake of enjoyment. It is mentally absorbing and healing because it invokes a spirit of play. With the mind absorbed, focused, and relaxed, stress is released, tension in the body is reduced, and pain diminishes.

It is important to regularly schedule entertainment into your life, whether it is listening to music or watching television at home, going to a movie or the theater, reading a book, or going to a sporting event.

Self-entertainment or entertaining others can add a challenging, creative dimension to entertainment, and may be even more fulfilling and rewarding than when you are simply being entertained as a spectator. Participating in the performing arts, in theater, dance, or music can serve this purpose. Painting, sculpting, sewing, making pottery, and many other activities may also qualify as self-entertainment because they engage the mind and are relaxing.

DANCING

To help ease the pain after my back surgery, I began moving my body to the beat of reggae music. I danced alone, too embarrassed that someone would see me. I was not dancing to entertain others, however, I was dancing for myself and it felt good!

The music took my mind off the pain and the dancing helped to stretch and strengthen the muscles in my feet, legs, and lower back. After several months, I saw that the pain in my back was lessening. I began to see that I was healing from the dancing, and every day I looked forward to it that much more. I saw also that my cardiovascular system and entire body were getting stronger from the movements, and I was reducing my weight as well. I incorporated a style similar to the aerobic dancing that is done daily in spas and health clubs. I listened to my body and let it guide me. I followed no structure or format other than listening to my body and the music.

From the dancing, with my muscles warmed up and relaxed, I moved into the pure stretching and stress management routines of yoga. The dancing helped set the tempo and tone for my body, putting me in the proper frame of mind to deal with the pain in my back in a constructive way.

If you have an ongoing back problem, I encourage you to start dancing to your favorite music. It helps if the music has some kind of beat and rhythm, but this is not essential. If you are in pain, start slowly with gentle movements and then build up gradually as you explore your body's limitations and your confidence increases. If you are embarrassed as I was, close the door and dance alone in front of a mirror. Try to build up to 30 minutes a day.

The smooth, graceful, and rhythmic movements of dancing help to heal your back by toning, stretching, and strengthening the muscles in your back and legs while improving the range of motion in your joints in a way that is gentle and therapeutic. The music adds to the enjoyment and fun.

When you dance, be inventive and spontaneous. Listen to your body; it will tell you how to move in a way that will feel good and will also be beneficial to your back. Any kind of dancing will do. Don't worry about getting the steps right. Just relax your body as you move. Remember, any kind of dancing will be beneficial to your health, as long as you listen to your body.

MUSIC

Music is considered one of the fine arts, a form of creative expression. But because music is also an energy, it can heal. For this reason, music is now considered a healing art. While the ancients have long since recognized this property of music, music therapy is now being offered in many major medical and hospital settings around the world. Because music can lift your spirits, it can help you overcome depression born of chronic pain. Mental institutions incorporate music therapy into their treatment regimens for this reason.

With its ability to stir emotions, music can also energize your body and mind, stimulating healing processes from deep within. When you listen to your favorite music, it can evoke fond memories of the past. It can release emotions, produce powerful mental images that reduce mental tension, relax the muscles in your body, and help to heal your back.

Because music can help you focus your mind on something beautiful and pleasing, it can make you forget about your pain. As Bob Marley said, "One good thing about music is it makes you feel no pain." It is healthier and often more effective than even strong narcotic pain pills. If you are lying in bed, unable to move because of your back pain, listening to music can help you relax, bear the pain, and pass your time more enjoyably until the pain subsides.

When listening to music for healing purposes, use a good quality stereo, CD, or tape player. Listen through headphones when you want to block out all outside sounds and focus exclusively on the music. Select your favorite music and adjust the volume so that it is full, but not too loud.

Because there are so many types of music from which to choose, here are just a few ways to use music to help you heal your back:

Music Therapy to Help Relax the Muscles in Your Back
Use this technique when you need to quiet your mind, relax your muscles and ease the pain in your back.

+ Listen to gentle, soft, and soothing music. Try to select music that incorporates the peaceful sounds of nature such as the falling rain, birds singing, or waves lapping up on the shore.

+ Lie down or sit in a reclining position in a comfortable chair so there is no pressure on your back.

+ Make sure you are comfortable and that you are alone in a quiet place where no one will disturb you for at least a half hour.

+ Breathe slowly and deeply while listening to help quiet your mind and relax the muscles in your back. Close your eyes and allow your body to relax as your mind focuses on the music.

+ Because this type of music can evoke certain peaceful visual images, let your mind be transported to wherever the sounds may take you.

+ After the music is over, stretch your body, breathe deeply, and take a few moments to savor the experience before getting up and moving on to your next activity.

Note: This type of music can also be used as background for your stretching and stress management regimen (see Chapters Four and Six).

Music Therapy to Lift Your Spirits and Energize Your Back

When you are tired, your spirits are low, or when you want to exercise, dance, or energize your body to help strengthen your back, try this music therapy technique:

✦ Select your favorite upbeat, rhythmic music. Make sure the music has a definite beat and the rhythm is not too fast or slow.

✦ Try to feel the rhythm of the music in your body. You can clap your hands or move your feet to see if you are in rhythm.

✦ With your mind as a passive observer, feel your body moving to the beat of the music.

✦ Remember, music is an energy and it can heal. Let the sounds and rhythm of the music energize your entire body, including your back.

Music can be healing for your back. It can also lift your spirits. Try to listen to some kind of music every day, even if it is the birds singing in the trees. Don't let a day pass without having music in your life, even if you are the one singing it.

SPORTS AND GAMES

Sports and games are good for your body and back because they provide movement and exercise. More important, however, when done properly, sports and games invoke a spirit of play, which can be healing for your mind as well as your body.

Your back shouldn't keep you from enjoying your favorite sports or games. If you like to participate in vigorous physical activity and your back is not currently strong enough to perform as it did in the past, you may need to modify your activities as your back heals. This requires an open mind and a flexible attitude. Remember *The Way of the Peaceful Warrior* by Dan Millman (see Chapter Five).

Sports and games were created to be fun activities, as well as to instill a healthy competitive spirit, but the win-at-all-costs attitude toward certain sports is unhealthy. Team sports instill camaraderie and a sense of togetherness which encourages intimacy, connectedness, and healing, but if they are too competitive, the pressure for top performance and winning takes the joy out of the sport. In team or individual sports, be careful of the competitive element. (For more discussion on sports and games, see Chapter Five.)

LOVEMAKING

Making love can be viewed as serious business, but if done right, it usually invokes a spirit of playfulness that can help to heal your back.

Nowadays, with people so busy and committed to demanding careers, time for intimacy and lovemaking is often sacrificed. After working all day and then coming home exhausted, other activities seem to take precedence, such as dinner, putting the kids to bed, finishing the chores around the house, watching television, and getting ready for bed. As this routine repeats itself day in and day out, it is easy to factor out lovemaking activities altogether. When this happens, intimacy disappears and relationships become strained. Is it any wonder that there are so many divorces and broken relationships?

It is important to cultivate a sense of sharing and intimacy in your relationships. We all need touching and affection, and when you share life with someone else, it takes on a richer and deeper meaning. Loving another human being uplifts the spirits and comforts the soul. When you express love through your own mind and body, touching with warmth, tenderness, and affection, you are opening the channels to receive the same love back. This love is a powerful healing force.

Many people with back problems feel physically inhibited for fear of straining or reinjuring their backs. This fear is totally unfounded. Making love, not as an end in itself, but rather out of a spirit of giving and sanctity, will find its own way and express itself gently and profoundly. It is the healing balm that will bring life into the back that is in pain.

The Healing Power of Humor

Norman Cousins, the well-known author, accidentally discovered the healing power of humor while battling a serious, life-threatening disease. In the 1960s, after visiting the Soviet Union during the famous SALT Treaty talks between John F. Kennedy and Nikita Khrushchev, Cousins contracted Ankylosing Spondylitis, a disease of the spine for which there was no known cure. After the diagnosis was made, he was admitted to a hospital where the only thing that could be done for him was to monitor his blood, give him pain medications, and wait for him to die.

Since he believed that he was dying, he decided to enjoy his last few months by watching comedies and comedians such as Candid Camera, Charlie Chaplin, the Three Stooges, Laurel and Hardy, and others. As he did, he discovered his condition improving. After 15 minutes of solid belly laughter, he found that he could sleep pain free for two hours. In addition, his blood reports showed signs of improvement. Within a year, he was totally cured. He then went on to write a best-selling book about his experiences entitled *Anatomy of an Illness*, which was on the *New York Times* bestseller list for 40 weeks.

Humor, comedy, and laughter embody the spirit of play perhaps better than anything else. When you are laughing and enjoying yourself, your mind is completely at ease. Studies are now showing that when you are laughing and having fun, powerful, beneficial chemicals such as endorphins, encephalins, neuropeptides, prostaglandins, and various hormones produced by the brain and endocrine system are released into the bloodstream to help promote healing.

It is important to cultivate a sense of humor and laughter in your life on a daily basis. It is not a luxury; it is essential to your health and especially for the healing of your spine. Start learning to be a jester. Think of funny stories. Reflect on what's funny in your life. Learn to laugh at yourself. Drop your seriousness. Seriousness is harmful to your health because it keeps you tense and tight, impacting on your back with extra stress and tension.

No matter what shape the world is in, sustained seriousness is never justified because it will make you sick, and if you are sick, your effectiveness in contributing to the good of this world will be compromised. In spite of atrocities committed against the people of Tibet, the exiled Dalai Lama maintains an amazing sense of humor while working to bring about peace.

Remember how you laughed as a child? Cultivate this spirit of playfulness in your everyday life. Seek out people who make you laugh, who make you feel good about yourself, with whom you can relax and be yourself.

Keep things light. An attitude of levity will spill over into your body, making you feel light, taking the burden of weight off your spine, relaxing tight muscles, and healing your back pain.

Start hanging around kids if you haven't already done so. Get into what they are doing, learn to play with them. Let them be your teachers. Follow them. They will show you how to enjoy life again. Their laughter, spontaneity, and sheer joy of living will inject healing energy into your tired and achy back.

A Final Word

To heal your back, you must learn to have fun and enjoy yourself. Playfulness begins as a state of mind, and being able to play is essential to your health and well being. Because it will help heal your back, taking time to play is not selfish, but rather the most responsible and unselfish thing you can do for yourself and others.

Please remember that the areas on play covered in this chapter are not comprehensive. Whatever makes you laugh, brings a smile to your face, makes you feel good inside, helps you forget about time and feel like a child, uplifts your spirits and helps take your pain away, will be healing for your back.

CHAPTER TEN

Back To Life: Emotional and Spiritual Lessons for Healing

I N THIS KEY CHAPTER, I want to share some of the deeper emotional and spiritual lessons my back has taught me as it has healed. The importance of these lessons has been reinforced through the experiences of my patients and the many exceptional healers with whom I have met and worked over the years. Because these lessons are universal, I believe they will be instrumental in the healing of your back as well.

If you are now suffering from back pain, or if you have suffered from back pain at any time in your life, you know how low your spirits can get as a result of the pain. Sustained pain can cause depression, which is incapacitating in itself.

When I became a chronic pain patient, I went into a terrible depression. I was unable to work or even muster a smile for three full years. On top of the depression, I was tired, worn out, cynical, and angry. I figured I had reached the end of the line and there was nothing more to live for. I was 36 years old.

In this state of despair and torment, I was convinced that I would never know joy or happiness again. I reasoned that joy and happiness were nothing but illusions anyway, proverbial golden carrots that God dangled in front of our noses to keep us motivated as we moved from the cradle to the grave.

The days passed slowly for me in this state of continuous pain and mental anguish, and as my spirits spiralled downward, I saw myself marking time, wondering if I would ever rejoin life again.

The image that came to my mind during this period was that of a river that had changed course. Once I was in the flow of things, in the midst of life. Now I was stranded on a deserted riverbank, watching from a distance as the river continued on its course without me.

It felt very lonely and empty to be taken out of the mainstream of life, like a race car driver in the midst of a race, forced to make a pit stop because of mechanical problems, or a pilot, grounded and having his wings taken away, knowing he'll never be able to fly again.

Fortunately, this difficult period is over and now life is different. With the pain and depression behind me, I am now back in the thick of things. I feel that my spirit is flowing like a swift and wide river towards the ocean of a greater destiny. I have regained my enthusiasm, a sense of purpose, and a renewed commitment to happiness and fulfillment.

Having been roasted by the hellfires of chronic pain, today I see that I am a much better person for having gone through the experience. Just as gold, in order to be purified, must first be superheated to remove the dross or impurities, so too I feel I have been purified by my pain. In my professional role as a physician, I feel I am now able to understand others' suffering in a way that I couldn't have possibly discovered through other methods. For me, pain turned out to be a gift and a genuine blessing.

If you are having ongoing back pain at this very moment, take solace in the fact that no matter how long you've been in pain, it is only temporary. Your pain cannot possibly last forever because nothing on this earth lasts forever. Apply the principles, strategies, and techniques in this book and your pain will soon go away. All that is required is effort, determination, and a little patience.

When you get discouraged, and we all do from time to time, go outside on a clear night and gaze up at the moon. Think of the moon's distance from the earth and the impossible task of a man landing on the moon. With effort and determination, the impossible became a reality. If effort and determination can land a man on the moon, they can also heal your back.

Your pain is teaching you a lesson, just as mine taught me. The greater the pain, the greater the lesson. Once you've learned the lesson, the pain will begin to let up and eventually it will disappear. As you conquer the mountain of pain one step at a time, wisdom will reward you at the end of your journey. You will realize that you are a better person for having gone through the experience.

Emotions and Your Health

Feelings, while processed, recognized, and often initiated by the brain, are actually experienced in the body. They are a clear example of how the mind and body are connected.

The link between emotions and physical health has been recognized since antiquity, yet only recently has science verified that a connection exists. Since your emotions are experienced as physical sensations in your body, being in touch with how you feel at any given moment will keep you in touch with your body. When you are in touch with your body, you can take better care of it and become healthier. Your body can also help you understand suppressed feelings and emotions.

The word emotion comes from the Latin, meaning to move out. An emotion is an energy that craves expression. Many of us were trained from early childhood to suppress and deny feelings and emotions. But research has shown this to be harmful to your health.

Emotions such as fear, anger, jealousy, and resentment, when internalized and suppressed, create toxic chemistry in your body, which can affect your back. These feelings produce tension in your system, which can cause the muscles in your spine to tense-up, contract, and even go into painful spasm. When you are tense and uncomfortable, you can be unpleasant to be around. As a consequence, you become isolated and lonely, which creates more stress and pain.

You can literally feel your feelings either in the area of your heart or gut if you take a deep breath, allow your mind to quiet down, focus on your body, and ask yourself how you feel. Listen to your body. It has its own intuitive wisdom and knows how you feel. Remember, feelings are located in the body.

Also, accept your feelings for what they are. Don't tell yourself to feel a certain way or not to feel a certain way. If you are angry, you are angry. If you are sad, you are sad. Some people think you should only feel joy or happiness, but there is no right or wrong when it comes to feelings. Feelings just are.

How to Get in Touch with and Express Your Feelings

Feelings are very powerful. Being in touch with how you feel, then learning how to communicate your feelings to others, is a critical step in the healing process. Instead of denying or suppressing your feelings, learn to express them.

First, learn to quiet your mind through the stress management techniques described in Chapter Six. This will make it easier to listen to your body. Then follow these simple, but effective steps:

1. Close your eyes and take a deep breath. Relax your shoulders. Relax your body. Take another deep breath and let your mind relax.

2. Once your mind has become somewhat relaxed, focus your awareness within.

3. Try to perceive a dominant sensation in the area of your heart or stomach, since these are the most common areas of the body where feelings can be experienced. Take your time. In the beginning, this may feel awkward. Don't worry. With a little practice, it gets easier. You may be feeling more than one sensation; that's okay. Just select the most dominant one.

4. Once you've identified a particular sensation in your body, search for a word that describes it. For example, the sensation you are feeling could be sad, angry, fearful, nervous, disappointed, lonely, happy, contented, peaceful, or something else.

5. Once you've identified the feeling, choose a way to express it that is comfortable for you. Remember that suppressing a feeling is a choice, but not a very healthy one. It is better to express the feeling, first to yourself, and then to others. This may seem awkward at first, but it will get easier with time and practice.

For example, if you are feeling angry, you may have a very good reason for feeling this way. Anger may be a healthy emotion for you to experience at this time, and suppressing it doesn't get rid of it. The anger remains within your body and can wreak havoc on your back.

You can release your anger by expressing it in a way that doesn't harm you or anyone else. There are many healthy ways to do this, such as simply stating, "I am angry!" You could also beat on a punching bag, or hit a pillow with your fists or a plastic baseball bat as you verbally express your anger. When you express anger in this way, you release it from your body, and if someone is around you they will know exactly how you feel.

Communicating feelings to another person, even negative feelings like anger, sadness, and disappointment, creates intimacy. Stuffing your feelings, and communicating only judgments about these feelings or about other people's feelings, creates separation and isolation, which can lead to stress. You can feel it in your body. If your back is sensitive, you can literally feel it tightening-up when you stuff a feeling, or when you are in the presence of someone else who is stuffing a feeling.

Because your feelings influence your health and your outlook on life, it is important to achieve a certain degree of mastery over them. You can do this only by being in touch with your feelings and emotions, not by suppressing them.

Keeping your mind calm by learning to relax and manage stress (see Chapter Six) will help you avoid stressful situations and focus on your natural sense of peace, contentment, and joy. Since emotional upset causes your back pain to increase, emotional mastery will help you avoid upsetting situations, calm your mind, and heal your back.

Spirituality and Your Health

Spirituality can be broadly defined as the ability to recognize a Higher Power in your life. It is the awareness of a divine hand in all of life and a sense of connection to all living things in the universe.

Spirituality depends on faith, that unique quality of the heart that holds things true even though unseen or not yet experienced. Every baby is born with abundant faith that erodes and wears away as we mature into cynical and embittered adults. With practice, however, faith can be renewed and restored.

Faith opens the heart to love. The greater the faith, the greater the capacity of the heart to give and receive love. Love strengthens and nourishes your spirit while enhancing its capacity to heal your back.

Love can appear mysterious. Because it lies beyond the realm of reason and logic, it has never been proven to exist by science. Yet love is the most practical and powerful force in the universe. It is the organic glue and foundational support that holds together families, societies, and all nations. Since the dawn of modern civilization, more books have been written on love than any other subject. Love makes the experience of life beautiful, sacred, and meaningful. Love is real, and is the most powerful healing force in the universe for anyone with back pain.

Emotions, Spirituality, and Healing

By learning to listen to the wisdom of your body and exploring the emotional roots of your back pain, you will discover the doorway to your own spirituality. The following lessons can help to guide you on your journey and expedite the healing of your back:

Avoid blaming yourself or others for your pain, whether it is physical or emotional.

When you blame others for the way you feel, you are giving away your personal power. And when you blame yourself, it is even worse. Wherever there is blame, there is punishment, and wherever there is punishment, there is pain. Pain creates anger and depression. Depression suffocates your spirit. Not blaming others, not blaming yourself, and not accepting blame from others will keep your energies focused on your own growth and healing.

Nobody is perfect. Everybody makes mistakes. I make more mistakes than most people I know, so I know you must make a few. Whatever imperfections you have, or whatever mistakes you have made, you must learn to forgive yourself.

Forgiveness, as with love, needs to be practiced each and every moment of the day until you can stop feeling guilty and blaming yourself. To forgive yourself for everything that you may have done wrong, for every person you feel you have disappointed, wronged, or injured, may take some effort, but it paves the way for self love. And love is always healing.

Don't live in fear and don't be afraid of your pain.

It has been said that all emotions can be reduced to a common denominator of two main emotions, fear and love. Fear causes anxiety, tension, stress, and anger, and these emotions all contribute to back pain through the mind-body mechanisms that we have discussed in earlier chapters. While fear causes pain, pain also causes fear. The two feed on each other in a destructive way. Fear blocks the flow of love and interferes with healing.

Many of our fears are imaginary. They are based on events from the past that we project into the future, and that usually have little to do with what is happening in the present moment. Learning to relax while practicing the stress management techniques described earlier will keep your mind focused in the present, while dispelling your fears.

Honor your pain as a teacher and a friend.

We often carry tremendous emotional baggage from our childhood and we aren't even aware of it. As we go deeper and deeper into the pain that is stored in our backs, it's like peeling the layers of an onion. We discover layers of emotional programming, that while buried, were previously sabotaging our healing.

Your pain is your guide through this maze of unconscious, suppressed emotions, as you peel back layers and bring new awareness to old, worn-out patterns of self-destructive behavior. Pain is the divine cosmic scalpel that heals you by cutting through these unconscious layers of suppressed emotions until you reach the core of the onion, the essence of your being, the foundation of who you really are. This is why pain needs to be honored as a teacher and a friend. Pain reminds you of who you really are.

Share your pain and you'll heal faster.

It takes courage to share your pain, but without risk, there can be no gain. Personally, I have benefitted tremendously from the process of sharing my pain. Once I found myself in a safe and nonjudgmental environment, I gave myself permission to share my painful childhood wounds and felt a huge burden lift from my back. It was a dramatic quantum leap in my development.

While we naturally assume that no one else wants to be burdened by our woes, the opposite is actually true. People feel closer to someone who is capable of baring their heart. The closeness creates intimacy and trust, and when they open up to you, you've helped to initiate their healing. It's an amazing process!

Learn to love your back.

No matter how bad your back is, how painful it is, or how many injuries or how much damage it has sustained, it is important to realize that your back is your best friend.

Your back is one of the most important parts of your body. When it goes out and you are unable to walk or move, you become aware of just how important it is. Until your back goes out, you usually take it for granted.

Your back is critical to your day-to-day functioning. It supports you while sitting, standing, and walking. It supports the weight of your head and your brain, the most important organ in your body. It protects and houses your spinal cord where all the nerves in your body originate. Not a single movement in your body can be done without affecting your back on some level.

Your back can tell you when you need to rest, when you need to slow down. Your back can tell you if you are eating the wrong foods, if you are under stress, if you are pushing too hard. This is extremely valuable information that can prevent you from getting sick in other ways that may be even more serious than a back problem.

You can choose to ignore your back for only so long. Soon, it will begin to talk to you. When you haven't been very good at listening, pain will come along to wake you up and refocus your attention on your back.

Learn to love your back as you would your best friend. Learn to care for it as you would anything else you love. Get to know what it needs to be happy. Try to understand it. Speak to it. Listen to it. Don't ignore it. Be open to continuous informational exchange and communication. Get to know what activities or modalities make it feel better, and what makes it feel worse. Understand its limitations. Nourish and nurture your back. Be kind to your back. Don't take it for granted. Accept it as it is without trying to change it. Work with your back. Cooperate with it. Help it to grow, to heal, to become strong. Don't overload it. Consult with your back as a partner in major life decisions that will have an impact on it. Take the time to massage it, keep it warm and comfortable. Exercise it. Find all the ways you can be good to your back. It is an ever-changing, constantly evolving, lifetime project.

When you are loving your back, you are really loving yourself because your back is one of your dearest possessions. A back that is loved reflects strength and health, flexibility and durability. When it is healthy and well cared for, your back will serve you faithfully over the course of a lifetime. It will carry and lift objects and help you move your body over great distances, on land, in the water, and in the air. Your back is there with you in the thick and thin of the countless activities you will experience in your lifetime.

Learn to love yourself. Love is the greatest healing force in the universe.

Love is your body's greatest source of strength and nourishment. As Dr. Bernie Siegel says, "Love is the most powerful stimulant known to the human immune system." Whereas fear creates disease and pain by causing tension in your system, love heals by creating peace and comfort. Love strengthens your spirit, relaxes your muscles, and soothes your nervous system. The most powerful medicine in the world is love, and it is found within each one of us.

All love begins within the individual. Since you can't give away what you don't have yourself, it is impossible to love others unless you love yourself first. I am not speaking of anything narcissistic or superficial, but of a profound love of self, something that needs to be practiced, learned, and experienced.

Self-love requires work. It means accepting yourself just as you are, with all the mistakes you've made in the past, and with all your present imperfections. It means not judging yourself while you learn to forgive yourself for your greatest transgressions. If you are used to beating yourself up, love of self can be hard work.

Your self-esteem and your ability to love yourself are connected and often reflected in the movement of your back. Do you have to bend over backwards for everyone? Do you have to bend over and pick up everyone else's trash or mess? These are questions with deeper, hidden meanings.

Sometimes you go out of your way for other people. This can be noble if love is your motive. But often you are doing this so other people will like you. You bend over backwards for other people or bow down to them because their opinion of you is crucial to your self-esteem. If they like you, you feel good about yourself. If they don't like you, you feel horrible.

Be yourself! You don't have to bend over backwards or bow down for anyone else. If someone does not appreciate you for who you really are, then that is their loss. It doesn't mean that something is wrong with you. It just means that they don't know you, they have their own problems, or their tastes are different from yours. Some people like lobster, others like steak.

When you love yourself, you will be kind and loving to your entire body, giving it the food it needs, proper rest, exercise, and stretching. You will not push your back beyond its capacity, and you will be sending kind and loving thoughts to your body through your mind to help create the harmonious chemistry that will allow your back to heal.

Develop healthy, loving relationships to nourish and support your back.

Relationships are your support systems in life. Relationships with your family, friends, neighbors, colleagues and coworkers all affect the health of your body and, ultimately, your back. Conflict in your relationships at home or in the workplace can cause extreme stress and tension in your system, which can trigger severe back problems. In fact, many patients suffer acute back problems right after a horrendous fight at home or in the midst of an ugly divorce.

Whether you choose to live alone while maintaining relationships with friends, neighbors, and families, or in a committed partnership with a significant other, clearly, "no man is an island," and healthy, loving relationships can serve as nourishing, spiritual support for your back.

In today's busy world, balancing work and family, playtime with quiet time, solitude and creativity, can be a real juggling act that ends up being extremely stressful. By listening to your body and consulting your back, you can learn to give to others while nourishing and taking care of yourself at the same time.

Develop a sense of unity and harmony in your life.

The human spirit is linked to a greater whole. When the mind is quiet and stilled of all its incessant mental activity, the opportunity arises to experience a sense of harmonious unity with all life. Experiencing a common unity constitutes a huge support network for your back. Meditation, spending time in nature, and learning to listen to the promptings of your own heart can help you experience this state of unity.

When you meditate or quiet your mind through the Back To Life stress management techniques (see Chapter Six), you will experience a place that is beyond thought. In this space, you will still be aware, still be conscious, and yet will know that you are a part of something bigger than yourself. In this center, you will discover your connection with all life. You will not feel lonely or separate.

Learn to acknowledge a Higher Power in your life.

Prayer can open a channel of communication for you to dialogue with the infinite and wise powers of our sacred universe. While many people pray when they are suffering or deeply troubled, prayer can also be appropriate for expressing feelings of gratitude and thanks. Prayer at either of these times can be highly therapeutic.

Many studies have been conducted demonstrating the efficacy of prayer in healing, and as a physician, I have witnessed its success enough times to recommend it as standard therapy to my patients. Prayer has been an instrumental factor in the healing of my own back.

Turning your burdens and worries over to a Higher Power relieves tension, and clears your mind and heart so you can receive from the universe your highest good.

Experience and appreciate the natural abundance in your life.

Because of the harmful effects of stress and tension on the spine, a fear of not having enough money to pay the bills and put food on the table for the family can be a real threat to the health of your back. What has been termed "poverty consciousness," or a sense of not having enough money and material things, can be a major source of stress for many back patients and was a factor in my own back troubles for many years.

As with depression, poverty consciousness comes from focusing on what you don't have, on what is missing in your life, rather than on what you do have. Rather than seeing your assets, you are consumed by your liabilities. It's a question of seeing the glass half empty rather than half full.

If a fear of poverty is the motivating factor in your desire to acquire large sums of money, then no matter how much money you have, it will never be enough. This will create constant tension in your life, which will create problems in your back.

You can overcome poverty consciousness by focusing on all your assets. You are worth much more than you think. Zig Ziglar, popular author and motivational speaker, tells a simple story that helps illustrate this point:

A woman who was given a medicine for her arthritis experienced a side effect that resulted in blindness. She was awarded one million dollars by the insurance company. Another woman broke her back in a plane crash and was awarded one million dollars by her insurance company. Betty Grable, the actress, was famous for her legs and had them insured for one million dollars each. So if you only consider your eyes, your back, and your legs, you're worth at least $4 million right there! Clearly, the best things in life are free!

When you see the vastness of the universe and the incredible beauty of the world in which you live, and when you see your body as a gift, you experience the natural abundance of life. When you enjoy the miracle of life in all its richness and fullness without fear, you create a state of ease in your body that will allow your back to heal.

If you focus on your assets in a spirit of gratitude, you will open yourself to the abundance of the universe, and over time you will discover that your back problems are only a vague memory.

= In Closing =

I AM GRATEFUL to have been able to share with you all that my back has taught me about life. I hope you will find this information helpful in bringing about your own healing. For easy reference, here is the essence of the Back To Life Program:

+ Remember the straw that broke the camel's back. You must look deeper than the last straw to understand your back problems.

+ Get to know your back. Review the anatomy. Learn to listen to your back and to your body. Remember the mind-body connection, and the important role of the back muscles in supporting your spine. Know how stress and mental tension affects your back.

+ Understand and get to know your pain. Discover its source. Embrace your pain as a friend and teacher. Don't fight, deny, or suppress it. Look for the deep emotional roots of your physical pain.

+ Stretch the muscles in your back and the rest of your body. Strengthen and tone your back muscles and the supporting muscles of the adjacent body parts.

+ Practice stress management strategies and techniques every day. Relax daily, and learn to quiet your mind with the breath. Practice meditation and mental imagery healing techniques.

✦ Watch what you put into your body. Avoid caffeine and nicotine. Eat healthfully. Develop good nutritional hygiene for your back.

✦ Mind and respect your back when you're at work. Remember not to push it too far. See your work as therapeutic. Don't be a workaholic.

✦ Develop a sense of humor, and take the time to play and smell the flowers. Spend time with children and cultivate intimacy in your relationships. Don't neglect your hobbies and extracurricular activities.

✦ Love your back and love yourself. Understand the connections between your emotions and your back. Get in touch with your feelings and learn to express how you feel. Remember your true self, and honor the challenge of your back as a doorway into the spiritual realm of your existence. Open yourself to the abundance of the universe.

Special Section:
Emergency Back Care

YOUR BACK HAS GONE OUT and you can't walk. You are experiencing the worst pain in your life. You can't sit. You can hardly turn over from your back to your belly. You're stuck on the floor. You're lucky if you can crawl. You can't sit on the toilet. You can't make it into the bathtub, let alone the shower. You're in a jam!

You're needed at work. Your family needs you. Your mortgage or rent is due and you have outstanding bills to pay.

The pain is incapacitating. Being incapacitated is stressful. The stress is causing more tension. The tension is tightening up your back muscles, creating more pain. You're in trouble. What are you going to do?

Follow these emergency back care instructions. You are free to pick and choose from the list, but I suggest you adhere to these interventions in the sequence given.

EMERGENCY BACK CARE INSTRUCTIONS

1. Do the Knees-Up relaxation technique (see Chapter Four, page 61).

Benefits: Takes the weight off the spine while supporting it. Relaxes the muscles in the back. This is generally the most comfortable position for a painful back.

✦ Lie on your back with your knees bent and your feet up on a chair or over a bed. A stack of pillows or blankets under your knees and lower legs can be used in place of a chair or bed.

✦ Lying in this position, practice deep relaxation by closing your eyes and watching the gentle movement of the breath as it flows in and out of your body. Feel the breath expanding into your stomach and abdomen as it enters into your body, and gently contracting your stomach and abdomen as it leaves your body.

✦ Relax all the muscles in your body.

✦ Continue to observe the flow of your breath as you focus your awareness on the movement of your stomach and abdomen. Do not try to control the rate or depth of the movement of your stomach and abdomen but rather try to allow them to move on their own. Relax your mind as well as your entire body.

✦ Remain in this position with your eyes closed for a minimum of 20 minutes. If you find yourself falling asleep, don't worry; it probably means that your body needs the rest. Repeat this deep relaxation several times a day until your pain ceases. Many people sleep in this position when their backs are painful.

2. **Do back breathing on your stomach** (see Chapter Four, page 75).

Benefits: Takes all the weight off the spine. Uses the breath to gently stretch and massage the deep, internal muscles of the spine. Relieves spasms and pain.

✦ Lie on your stomach, placing a pillow or two under your hips for support if you need it.

✦ Adjust your body until you find a comfortable position, turning your head to one side and resting it on your hands. Adjust your legs, hips, back, arms, shoulders, neck, and head so that the muscles in these parts are relaxed.

✦ Breathe slowly and deeply, feeling the gentle rising and falling of your stomach and abdomen as the breath flows in and out of your body.

✦ As the breath comes into your body and expands your entire abdomen, chest, and rib cage, feel the muscles in your back gently stretch and expand. Slowly deepen the movement of the breath, allowing it to expand, stretch, and massage the tight and painful muscles in your spine.

✦ Breathe like this for 10-15 minutes every 1-2 hours while you are awake. Remember not to hold your breath or force or strain in any way.

3. **Do the Cobra Arching stretching technique** (see Chapter Four, page 75, then page 77).

Benefits: This opens the spine, helps to take the weight and pressure off the spinal column and discs, elongating and stretching the muscles of the spine and hips.

✦ Lying on your stomach, gently raise your chest and head until you feel an arching sensation in your back.

✦ Rest the weight of your head on your hands and elbows if you are able, or place a pillow or two beneath your chest for support.

✦ From this position, try to push up all the way, using your hands and arms to support the weight of your upper body.

✦ With your chest off the floor, breathe deeply, feeling the full expansion of your stomach and abdomen as the breath flows into your body. As your stomach and abdomen expand, feel the gentle pulling sensation on your lower spine. Feel the spine extending and stretching as you breathe in this position.

✦ Relax your lower spine.

✦ Squeeze and tighten your buttocks muscles and then relax them, repeating this tensing and relaxing of the muscles for as long as you are able to maintain this position.

✦ If your back pain is off to one side, try to stretch away from the pain, using your shoulder and hip on the side of the body where you are experiencing the pain to lengthen the spine on that side.

✦ Try to maintain this position for at least 1-2 minutes.

✦ Do not force or strain. If you become tired or need to rest for any reason, slowly lower your chest and head down to the floor, close your eyes, observe the movement of your breath, and relax.

✦ Wait a few moments, then once again attempt to come up into this position with your chest and head raised.

✦ Repeat this stretch 10 times every hour while you are awake. If it is too painful, and you feel you can't do it at all, go back to relaxation and back breathing and attempt this the following day.

4. **Eat lightly and drink plenty of fluids.** See Chapter Seven for additional dietary and nutritional advice.

5. **Avoid all stimulants, including caffeine and nicotine.** See Chapter Seven for additional dietary and nutritional advice.

6. **Avoid sitting, since sitting is the hardest position for the spine.**

7. **Avoid prolonged standing.**

8. **Don't bend forward for 3-4 days.**

9. Avoid driving and moving around too much.

10. Keep your mind positive and stay busy with reading, listening to music, watching movies (especially comedies), and other fun and uplifting activities. Don't allow yourself the time to brood or become despondent.

11. Rest and relax.

12. Call your relatives, family members, and friends for support.

13. Take a jacuzzi, sauna, steam, or warm bath.

14. Try massage, physical therapy, or both.

15. Apply either heat or ice to your back, whichever works best for you. (I prefer heat!)

16. Apply your favorite heat balm. (I like Tiger Balm.)

17. Decide where you want to sleep and what will feel better for your back: a bed or the floor?

18. If after several days your back is not improving, consider one or more of the following alternative therapies if they are available in your area: massage, physical therapy, chiropractic, yoga therapy, acupuncture, biofeedback, osteopathic manipulation, myofascial release, Reiki, healing touch, reflexology, homeopathy, Lomi lomi, (traditional Hawaiian massage), Ayurveda, and anything else that is safe, gentle and effective, and in which you have confidence. The bottom line is that you should use what works for you and what you believe will help you. This includes prayer and the power of positive thinking.

19. Consider making an appointment with your physician or

health care provider if your pain is not going away after one or two weeks. He or she may prescribe medication to relax the muscles temporarily and ease the pain and/or order a test to further evaluate your pain.

When you feel the pain starting to ease up, go back to the beginning of this book and read it in its entirety. If you follow the Back To Life Program faithfully, you will never need emergency back care again!

Recommended Reading

Anderson, Bob. *Stretching*. London: Pelham Books.

Benson, Herbert, M.D. *The Relaxation Response*. London: Fount Publishers.

Borysenko, Joan. *Minding the Body, Mending the Mind*. Harrow: Publishers Marketing Services.

Bresler, David. *Free Yourself from Pain*. New York: Simon and Schuster.

Catalano, E.M. *The Chronic Pain Workbook*. Oakland, California: New Harbinger.

Chopra, Deepak, M.D. *Quantum Healing*. New York: Bantam.

Cousins, Norman. *Anatomy of an Illness*. New York: W.W. Norton.

Cousins, Norman. *Head First: The Biology of Hope*. New York: E.P. Dutton.

Dossey, Larry, M.D. *Healing Words*. San Francisco: Harper.

Goleman, Daniel and Joel Gurin. *Mind Body Medicine*. Yonkers, New York: Consumer Reports Books.

Hay, Louise. *You Can Heal Your Life*. Middlesex: Eden Grove Editions.

Kabat-Zinn, Jon. *Full Catastrophe Living: Using the Wisdom of Your Body and Mind to Face Stress, Pain and Illness*. New York: Doubleday/Dell Publishing Group.

Kuvalyananda, S. *Yoga Therapy*. Faridabad, India: Government of India Press.

McKenzie, Robin. *Treat Your Own Back*. Waihanae, New Zealand: Spinal Publications.

Monro, Robin, R. Nagarantha, and H.R. Nagendra. *Yoga for Common Ailments*. New York: Fireside Books.

Rossman, Martin, M.D. *Healing Yourself*. New York: Pocket Books.

Sarno, John, M.D. *Healing Back Pain*. New York: Warner Books.

Scaravelli, Vanda. *Awakening the Spine*. San Francisco: Harper.

Schatz, Mary Pullig, M.D. *Back Care Basics*. Berkeley: Rodmell Press.

Siegel, Bernie, M.D. *Love, Medicine, and Miracles*. London: Arrow Books.

Siegel, Bernie, M.D. *Peace, Love, and Healing*. London: Arrow Books.

Tobias, Maxine and Mary Stewart. *Stretch and Relax*. London: Dorling Kindersley.

Weil, Andrew, M.D. *Spontaneous Healing*. New York: Knopf.

White, Augustus, M.D. *Your Aching Back*. New York: Simon and Schuster.

Index